NO QUICK FIXES

A Fitness Journey for the Real World

NO QUICK FIXES

A Fitness Journey for the Real World

Lindsay B. Nauen, MBA
and
Keith Gosline, ACSM EP-C, CMAT, CKTP

Nauen Retirement and Educational Services, LLC
ISBN 978-0-692-16102-9

First Printing 2018

Edited by Russell Resources LLC, *www.russellresourcesllc.com* or *www.writer.mn*
Designed by Sue Stein

Cover image © 2011 Lynn M Jonson with Glass Moon Photography
Back cover and images pages 30, 35, 70, 87 and 99 © 2018 Sue Lund Photography
Images pages 22, 67 and 68 © 2018 Grupa Portrait Studio
Chart, page 46 © 2018 PostNet, St. Paul, MN

Medical Disclaimer: This book is designed to provide helpful information on the subjects discussed and is not a substitute for professional medical treatment or diagnosis. The content in this book is for informational purposes only. The author, editor and publisher assume no responsibility for the accuracy of information in this book. You are encouraged to confirm and review with your physician information regarding medical conditions or treatment.

Table of Contents

FOREWORD

Lindsay Nauen met with me for an initial evaluation on January 23, 2006. She was referred to me because of her health issues and personal health concerns. One of her major concerns was how she could enjoy life to its fullest with her current health status. Lindsay told me when she traveled with her husband, she had to stay in the hotel. She could not walk more than one block before she was exhausted. Needless to say, Lindsay was ready to explore options and find a trainer she could work with safely and effectively. I dare say that she wasn't really sure what fitness could mean for her, but she was determined to find out.

As an ACSM-certified exercise physiologist (ACSM EP-C), certified massage therapist (CMT) and former post-secondary biomechanics, anatomy and physiology instructor, my scope of practice includes working with the medical conditions Lindsay was experiencing on a daily basis. I specialize in testing, customized training, myoskeletal alignment therapy, kinesio taping as a certified kinesio taping practitioner (CKTP), corrective exercise training for dysfunctional motor patterns, functional exercise to improve daily living activities and habits, and progressive sports performance rehabilitation, periodization and macrocycle training for sports performance.

Initially, my vision focused on giving Lindsay the confidence and compassion she needed. A skillful trainer understands there is no place for judgment. You need to be empathetic and to open up possibilities where there seemed to be none before. Lindsay says that I made it possible for her. That's the rewarding side of my job—to show people how to attain goals and create a new future they never knew were possible for them.

As we worked together, we became a team striving for consistent and progressive results. I outlined what we would work on, why it was important and guided her throughout the process of change. I recognized that she was intelligent and tenacious enough that she would value and honor the commitments she would make.

We started slowly, yet confidently, toward the larger goal of good health and fitness. I did not overwhelm her with the big picture or what was in store in the future. Rather, we focused on what she could do, not what she couldn't do. This was clearly the best way to inspire and instill confidence in each small victory as we worked through her fitness program.

I believe strongly that to be successful and build confidence and self-esteem, a program must be a positive, rewarding experience. Everyone needs rewards. We set expectations so the routines would feel good and set micro goals for every workout. I wanted Lindsay to understand that exercise is not something to fear, and that it could be an integral part of her life—and something to enjoy.

Lindsay began by committing to only three minutes each day—on the stairs, one stair or step bench—which was something she knew she could do. We gradually worked up to greater achievements, always taking into account her weight, history of polio, high blood pressure and metabolic factors. She learned to climb the mountain, one step at a time.

Exercise and lifestyle systems are more effective when they are achievable, modifiable and fun. When the exercise or program is not enjoyable, most people will not want to do it. They will quit. Lindsay had a consistent level of commitment which put her in the 10% of the population who would follow through with a plan. Having a positive, unwavering attitude and a knowledgeable, dedicated trainer completed the success formula. Lindsay learned to value herself and bring her 'A' game every day. I am proud of the work Lindsay has done, and it brings me joy when I see her self-assured smile.

This book is a powerful testament to Lindsay's hard work and belief that you can make positive changes as certainly as you can remain in a less productive routine. It took time, but Lindsay learned how to create a habit of movement and functional exercise. Her life has been forever changed by the new possibilities she has created for herself.

I am sincerely pleased to have played a role in her transformation, and that I can continue to guide her on her journey. My hope is that Lindsay's book will make a profound impact in the lives of others. Read on and see how inspiring one St. Paul woman can be!

Keith Gosline, ACSM EP-C, CKTP, CMAT
Fitness trainer and owner
Gosline-MAPP, SRL
Santo Domingo, Dominican Republic

INTRODUCTION

Why I Wrote This Book

This book is written for all those who need a fitness journey. Your journey could be to lose weight, stop smoking or improve your health. We are all on a life journey; why not be on a healthier one?

My fitness journey started in 2006. Now I have lost over 160 pounds and have become an athlete. During these 12 years, I have met people who are interested in my story. Family and friends have said I am inspiring and they could never have done what I did. I disagree. We all have the ability to change our lives, but it takes determination and a support team of family, friends and professionals.

The subtitle of *No Quick Fixes* is *A Fitness Journey for the Real World*. I have come from less to more. From less activity to participating in over 175 events. From morbidly obese to a healthy athlete. From a small life of work and little energy to a more complete life where I do not yet know all that I can and will accomplish. Two consistent messages my trainer tells me are: 1) you can manage your stress and fears or be managed by your stress and fears, and 2) my potential is always changing; therefore, my "best" is always changing too.

I have learned to believe in myself and my ability to change. I have learned the importance of support from professionals as well as family and friends. I have learned to set goals that are measurable, obtainable and flexible.

I have learned many lessons, including the importance of balance, the need for support, having a positive perspective and an effective attitude. I have learned the joy of celebration.

Now I also enjoy being healthy and active when I travel. Travel becomes an opportunity to sample new fresh fruits, vegetables and fish and participate in various types of enjoyable activities.

My family has changed for the better too. My husband, Richard, has lost weight and learned that he is an athlete also. Now, besides participating in triathlons with me, he runs several half marathons each year. We also enjoy at least one destination event in the winter to a warmer place than Minnesota. We have completed running events in California, Florida, South Carolina and Georgia.

I will never go back. The obese person I was has been transformed by this journey. I have more confidence and recognize that, if I can lose weight and keep it off, there is likely much more that I can accomplish. I have also transformed my attitude. I now focus on what I can do, not what I can't. Another change has been to realize that I will accomplish my goals. I now think in terms of when! —not if.

In this book, you will learn about my journey, read about the lessons I have learned, and gain some strategies to help you on your journey. As I have learned:

Because I can.
Because I like it.
Because it's good for me.

SECTION ONE

MY JOURNEYS

Chapter 1

My Fitness Journey

At the beginning of 2006, I was a middle-aged, sedentary accountant. My idea of exercise was going for a stroll when the weather was good. It was now winter in Minnesota, and I had no plans for exercise. A few years earlier, my doctor had put me on appetite suppressant medicine, and I had lost about 50 pounds; but weighing in at 296, I was still morbidly obese.

My accounting business had been growing steadily over the past two years, and I had been working

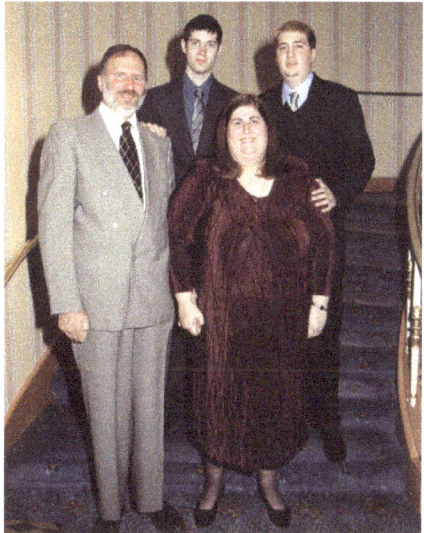

Our 25th anniversary picture

with a life coach, Jeanne Heald, to manage the growth. She suggested that I hire a personal trainer so that when spring came I would be able to do more walking.

As I was sedentary and not that familiar with exercise programs or trainers, I had no knowledge about how to find a personal trainer. I asked for advice from Sarah Kennedy, a member of my networking group, Business Network International (BNI), who had been a personal trainer. Sarah said the most important quality was for the trainer to have a designation from the American College of Sports Medicine (ACSM). She knew of one in BNI: Keith Gosline.

I called Keith and met with him on January 23, 2006. He did a Fitness Assessment and asked for a doctor's medical release and prescription letter before we began training on January 30th.

Today, I am an endurance athlete who has participated in over 175 events, including running in 5Ks (3.1 miles) and half marathons (13.1 miles), duathlons that include biking and running, and triathlons which are events that include swimming, biking and running.

In this book, I will tell you about my fitness journey and what I have learned. I will also include some of the life lessons I have learned that have given me the tools to be successful once I decided to become fit.

2006

When I started working with Keith Gosline, an ACSM EP-C (certified clinical exercise physiologist) who had also trained other obese, post-menopausal women, the focus was to get moving and raise my heart rate. I started with three minutes of aerobics a day, and I needed to work out every day. He asked for two things: that I add a minute a day every week and, when I got to 30 minutes a day, I could have a day off. It took me from January until April before I achieved that goal!

At that point, his training was purchased in 10-hour blocks. After 10 hours, I had not learned all the basic stretches, so he signed me up for another 10. However, he would not sign me up for a third set unless I had a fitness goal.

What was a fitness goal? I had never had a fitness goal in my life. Keith did not give me any suggestions. It was entirely up to me. After a week of agonizing, I asked very tentatively if running a 5K could be a fitness goal. After receiving a nod from Keith, I chose a 5K race that took place in August during the Minnesota State Fair.

This began my training for my first event. We trained in a beautiful St. Paul park, and I started running for 30 seconds and walking for two minutes. I slowly worked my way up to about half running and half walking for most of our one-hour sessions.

Just before the race, I had lost enough weight to be able to balance on a bicycle. My brother-in-law Jeffrey Burton took me shopping, and I found a fabulous Raleigh bike. Keith said it was okay to ride, but not to go too fast. With that advice in mind, I rode so slowly that I fell and bruised my knee. Keith still kids me about calling him, asking what to do and then insisting that at our next session he look at my knee. (Think of a child with an "owie!")

My First Race: The Rice Street Mile

As I was preparing for my first 5K, a colleague suggested that I practice with a short race. The only race shorter than the 5K was a one-mile race, the Rice Street Mile. So, on a 90° July day, I lined up with other women to run one mile on Rice Street, an urban street near my home.

What I didn't realize was that people who run one-mile races are sprinters. They are fast! Everyone took off, and I chugged along while people on the sidewalk cheered me on. The first quarter mile seemed to take forever although I finished the race in 16 minutes, 3 seconds. In fact, some of the women who had already finished came back and ran with me to the finish line. This was my first experience of the power of an informal support team. I had finished my first race and, to date, have participated in over 175 events.

My First 5K: The Milk Run

Finally, it came—August 27, 2006. It was called the Milk Run because it

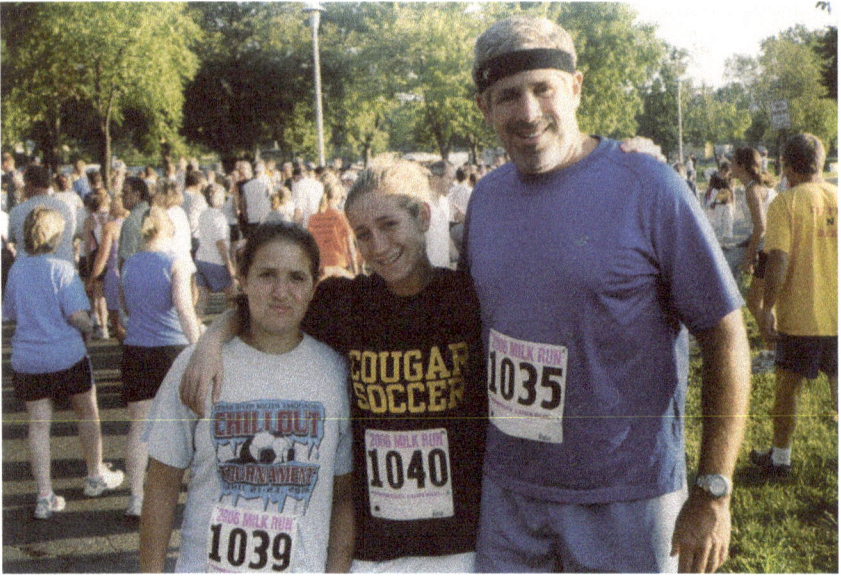

2006 Milk Run
Support team smiles from Hannah, Rachel and Charlie Nauen

took place during the Minnesota State Fair. Not only was I running in it, but I joined my brother, Charlie, and my nieces Rachel and Hannah. I started following my plan of partial walking and partial running, and when I got to the first mile, my massage therapist at the time, Dave Peterson, was calling out the times. I was averaging just over 18 minutes per mile.

I ran through the neighborhood adjacent to the fairgrounds, ran and walked through the University of Minnesota Saint Paul campus and finally back to the fairgrounds. During the last half mile, a mother and daughter running together would pass me, then I would pass them. Finally, with the end in sight, I put on a burst of speed and crossed the finish line. It felt great!

I had met my goals. I had completed my first 5K run, and I wasn't last! My time was 57 minutes and 12 seconds. At the finish line were Jeanne, Keith, Ben, Charlie, Rachel, Hannah and my husband, Richard. It felt good to see their smiles and pride in my accomplishment.

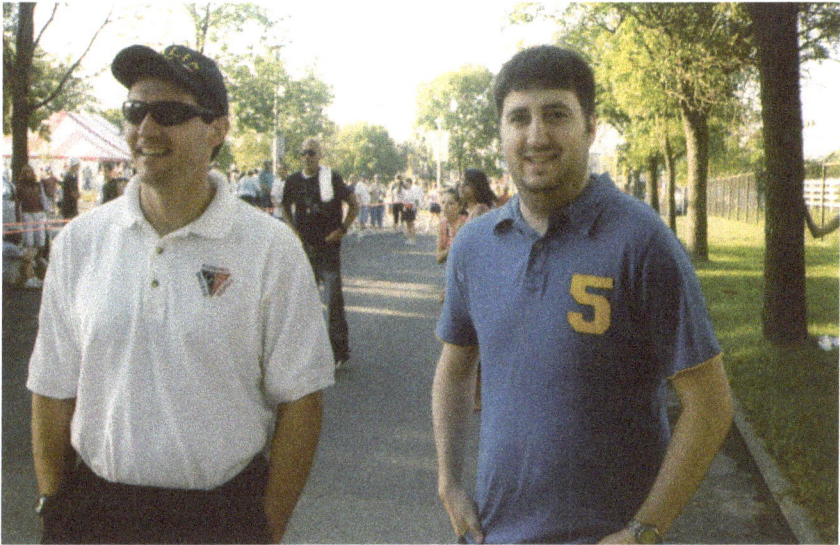

Cheering section: Keith Gosline and Ben Weil

Remainder of 2006

That fall, I did about one 5K per month, and Keith told me that swimming would improve my running, so we met at the local YWCA for my first session. I was very nervous about my trainer seeing me in a bathing suit. I still wore one with a skirt. When we met on the pool deck, I felt more comfortable when he said it was very colorful. Soon, I graduated to a tank style.

As I enjoyed riding my bike, leaning to swim better and running 5Ks, Keith brought up a new goal for me to train for triathlons. I learned that a sprint triathlon is a shorter event that includes a swim of ¼ to ½ mile, a bike ride of 11–15 miles, and most often, a 5K run. I was interested, and Keith told me I would need to train five hours per week for six months to get ready for my first event. Never in the history of triathlons did someone train so much for a sprint triathlon!

Periodization Plan

Keith provides further education, guidance and support through a progressive and personal training plan called a Periodization Plan. A Periodization Plan is a comprehensive endurance training schedule to prepare me to be at my peak—peak is my highest level of fitness and performance—at the time of an athletic event such as a 5K, marathon or triathlon. Each week, I exercise a certain number of minutes in my five heart rate zones and do exercises for muscular endurance or power. Keith always has me working on my flexibility as well.

Flexibility is the key element for all other areas in my fitness and performance training. Keith creates the periodization plan based upon various past and present considerations such as my prior medical history, fitness testing, exercise history and customized heart rate zones. Each week, I also work out in different heart rate zones for different amounts of time based on the cycle. A cycle is four weeks, so when I'm training for an Olympic triathlon for six months, I have six cycles in my Periodization Plan.

In general, the names of cycles are classified as: base, intensity, peak and race. If I am training for a triathlon, swimming is the fewest number of minutes, running is second, and biking is the most.

Periodization training is challenging, yet fun, and every plan is unique. Since Keith continually demonstrates to me that my best always changes, each Periodization Plan changes as well. No two are the same. In addition, the number of hours I train every week can be fixed or variable. For example, for the first eight years, I did fixed periodization plans (every week training for the same number of total hours or minutes per week), but in 2015 and 2016, I did the first 13 weeks fixed and the second half variable. Finally, in 2017, my entire periodization was variable as I trained for Olympic distance triathlons only. The Olympic length is also called the International Distance Triathlon. It consists of a .93-mile swim, a 40K bike ride and a 10K run.

Group Class

Since it was now winter, I began taking indoor cycling classes at the YWCA that I had joined. This was my first experience in a group setting. The instructors were always so encouraging of my efforts and several of them have become members of my informal support team.

2007

In February of 2007, I did my first destination 5K in Palm Springs. It was motivating and encouraging to understand that I could not only participate in hometown events but could also make it a vacation highlight. I've since learned to find interesting events in other cities to add some physical activity and enjoyment to my travel plans, and it's become something fun for the whole family.

All the determination and periodization training paid off when I ran my first triathlon in Alexandria, Minnesota in May 2007. It was 600 yards in a pool, followed by 12 miles of biking and a run of just under three miles. My husband, Richard, my best friend, Mickey, and Keith were all there to see me finish. I had Keith pin a dolphin pin on my shirt to commemorate finishing my first tri.

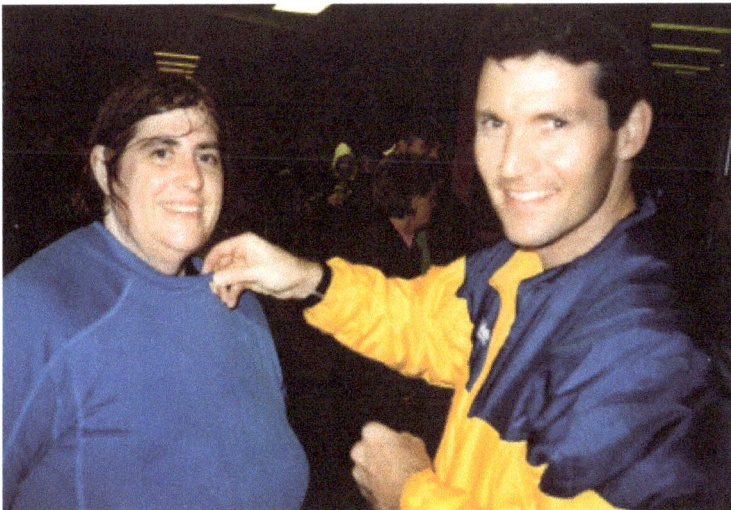

Keith pinning me after one year of training and my first tri

That year, I finished two more triathlons, each time training with a periodization plan.

My First Triathlon

Let me give a deeper description of my first triathlon.

Triathlon is an endurance sport that consists of three events: swimming, biking and running. My first tri was a 600-yard swim, a 12-mile bike and a 2.8-mile run.

Alexandria, Minnesota is a great venue for the beginning triathlete because the swim is in a pool. (Most Midwest triathlons are held in lakes in the summer.) In the pool, you swim 24 lengths with someone holding cards to keep track of how many laps have been completed. Richard was my card holder. There were eight lanes in the Discovery Middle School pool.

After the swim, I dressed in biking clothes and ran outside to the transition area. This is where all the bikes are racked, and bike shoes are set up. Running shoes, visors and water bottles are in another place in the same general area.

I ran my bike through transition, mounted it and started pedaling. It

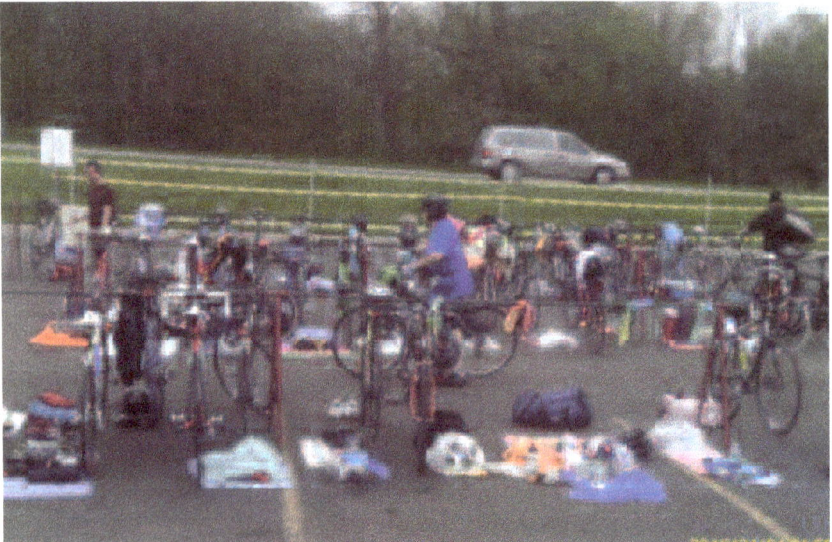

Transition Area

was cloudy and rather cool in Alexandria as I set out on the 12-mile bike ride. After one hour and 13 minutes, I was back in transition to switch to the run.

I put on my race bib, drank some water and was off for the run (which I mostly walked). As I approached the last grass strip to the finish line, there was Keith with his golf umbrella, urging me to the finish line. I had done it—my first tri—in a total time of 2:37:47.

Swim 23:17
T1 (Transition) 4:49
Bike 1:13
T2 (Transition) 2:38
Run 49:03
Total 2:37:47

The plan was to finish two more triathlons that summer, about six weeks apart. For each triathlon, Keith calculated a new periodization training plan. I finished the MinneMan on July 5th with a total time of 2:36:45. Jerry McNeil was the announcer, and he has become an additional member of my support team. He has often talked about my weight loss at subsequent

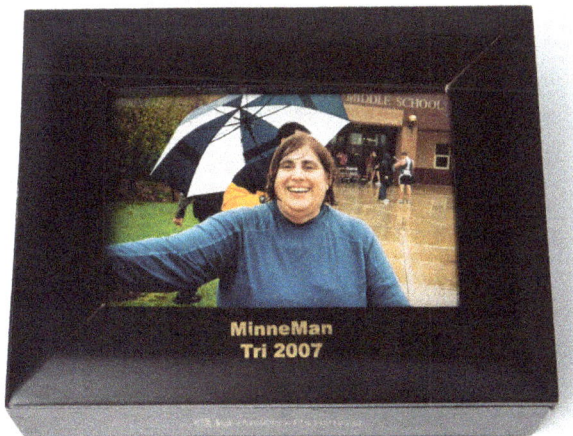

This photo is me at the end of my first triathlon (joyous!).
The box commemorates my second triathlon.

events. This was the start of a ten-year streak of "No DNFs" (Did Not Finish) that remained unbroken until my 151st event and my first triathlon in 2016. That's when I fell off my bike and couldn't finish because the bike frame was bent.

October of 2007 offered me another opportunity for a destination event while in Las Vegas vacationing with my son Ben. While my son slept in after a busy day in Las Vegas, I decided to run a 5K. This was my first time participating in an event without an informal support team. It was fun to be part of a group of runners in a new place, and again, I found out how much fun it can be to add events to vacations.

2008

In 2008, I needed a new goal for running events, which was to try some longer distance races. I did two 6Ks, an 8K and a 10K. I was able to compete in these longer events because I continued to train and lose weight. My first 10K was quite a challenge, but again, I finished. This time, I was last because I walked/ran 20-minute miles. It was my slowest pace of any race, but it was a great sense of accomplishment to finish that 6.2 miles!

To celebrate this achievement, I had a pin made with a roadrunner surrounded by 6K-8K-10K 2008. On the back, I had *Determination* inscribed because it takes a lot of training and determination to complete longer distances.

The types of training I did with Keith also evolved. I started with aerobics and strength training using bands. Later, he added fitness cuffs to the strength training mix.

Keith also wanted to add some calisthenics, but I wanted nothing to do with that. In fact, I told him that I didn't want to pay him to teach me something I didn't want to do! You may ask why. It was because in the early 1960s, as a response to the successful Soviet Sputnik launches, the National Defense Education Act was passed which affected physical education as well as science education. I had grown up being subjected to horrible calisthenics training to music. *Chicken Fat* was a fast-paced song with no instruction. It was written by Meredith Wilson of *Music Man* fame to get American children in shape and prepared to fight the Soviets. I had to do it marching in place to a militaristic tune. How horrible is that?

Keith was undeterred by my attitude and a few weeks later said again that it was time to add calisthenics to my routine. I plaintively asked, "Isn't strength training enough?" He educated me on the benefits of calisthenics which uses several muscles together at the same time. After making him listen to *Chicken Fat*, I started a new phase of training.

Now, I enjoy calisthenics such as jumping jacks, up-downs, dips, windmills and helicopters. Thankfully, Keith has never played *Chicken Fat* during a session!

All-Women Events

In 2008, I did a destination event in Seattle, participating in a triathlon with my cousin Viki. This was an all-female event sponsored by Danskin. Women-only events are different than mixed events in several ways. There is less emphasis on competition and more emphasis on the opportunity to participate. Also, there is more support, especially during the swim portion, where there are swim buddies with swim noodles to help those who are fearful in the water.

I have participated in a few other all-female events, including the Iron Girl Duathlon in Bloomington, Minnesota.

Another popular all-women event is the YWCA of Minneapolis sprint triathlon that takes place in August. This is one event where I am certain to find participants who are older than I am!

2009

In 2009, I tried a new event, a duathlon, composed of just running and biking. I did it as a relay with my husband. He did the running and I did the biking. It was a fun spring activity that we could enjoy together.

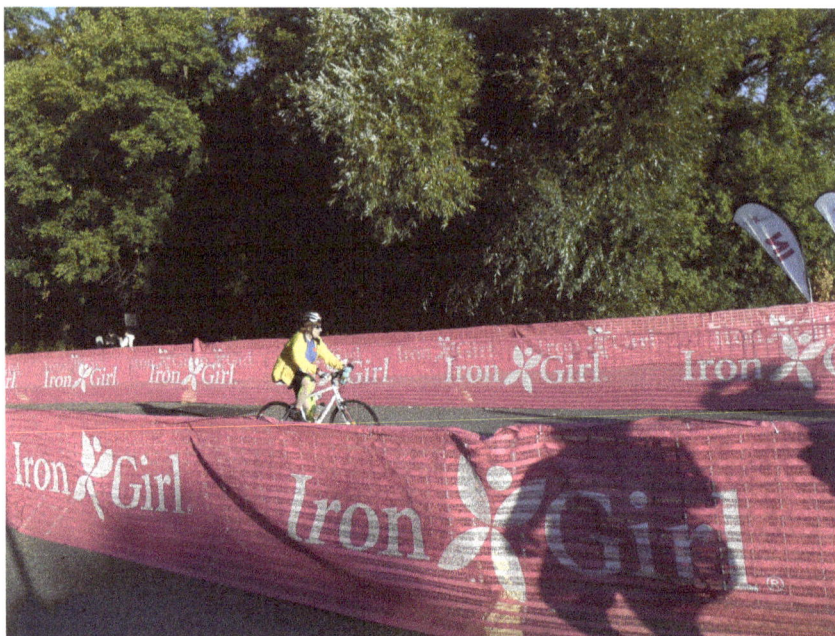

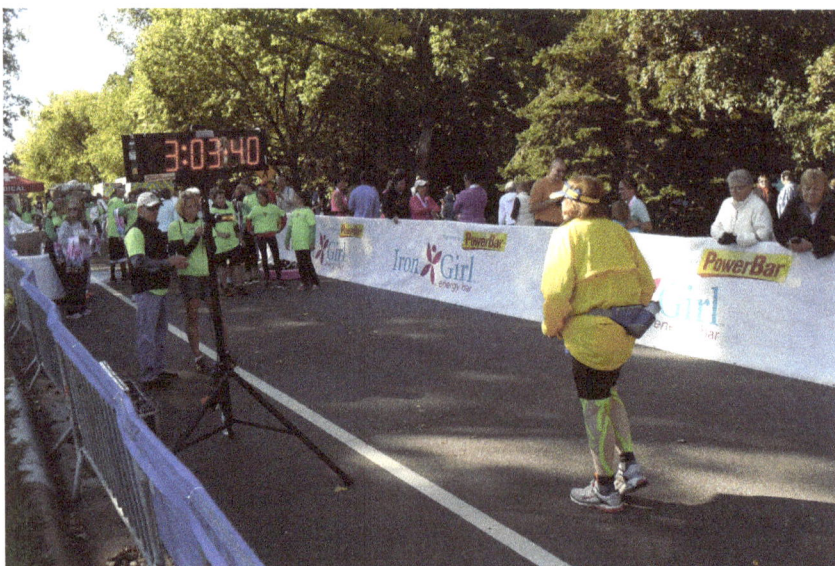

Minneapolis Iron Girl Event

I also did some triathlons in Fairmont and St. Paul, Minnesota with a friend. It was fun to train with a person who was similar in ability.

Finding training partners has been a challenge for me. Most middle-aged people have been active for years and already have their regimens and routines established. Since I am basically a shy person, it has been difficult for me to find training partners.

For biking, I joined some meet-up groups with enjoyable activities. Most of the running groups are for people training for marathons, who are just too fast for me. My favorite group activity has been the indoor cycling classes at my local YWCA.

2010

This year, I did some sort of event in every month except January. I did an indoor triathlon in March, but it is not an event I repeated. An indoor triathlon consists of swimming in a pool, riding a stationary bike and running on a machine or around an indoor track.

Also, this was the year that Richard started joining me in triathlons. He was tired of watching me and waiting for me to finish. He wanted to join me in the fun! Keith and Richard trained together in a local park in Falcon Heights, Minnesota to improve Richard's technique and perspective on running. He was now properly trained in the basics and ready to safely accomplish his goals. Keith started providing manual therapy and fitness training with Richard and encouraged him to begin walking and running.

With his lack of flexibility as well as a medical condition he has lived with since birth, Richard did not believe he could run. His lower leg bones, bones below the knee, are twisted; therefore, when he stands with his knees and feet together, his feet turn to the outside or diagonal to about 45 degrees. This puts a lot of stress on the inside of the ankles, knees, hips and back when running or biking.

I am so proud of Richard. He has overcome many obstacles and now has his own fitness journey. He has really accomplished a great deal, and I am excited to see what more he can do!

I finished four triathlons and really enjoyed another duathlon. This duathlon, the Iron Girl mentioned earlier, was a women-only event which again was run, bike, run in a local suburban park.

I also finished nine running events, mostly 5Ks and one 8K, the same one I had completed in 2008 and 2009.

2011

In the winter of 2011, my husband and I did our first destination event together in Hilton Head, South Carolina. I did a 5K, and Richard did the 10K. I also finished my first Olympic distance triathlon. To train for this, I participated only in longer distance triathlons in June and July.

An Olympic distance triathlon, also called the International Distance, is based on the lengths at the Olympics: 1500-meter (0.9-mile) swim, 40K (24-mile) bike and a 10K (6.2-mile) run. I was nervous that August morning at Weaver Lake in Maple Gove, Minnesota, a suburb about 30 minutes from

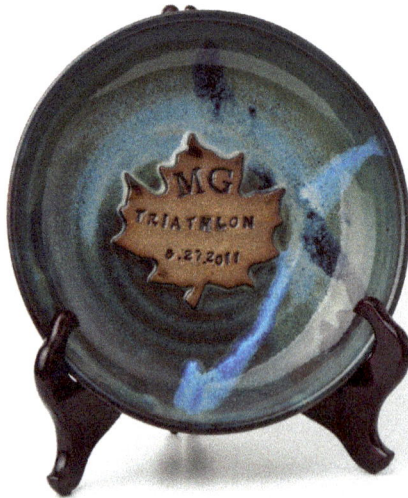

Handmade plate for Age Group Winner in my first Olympic triathlon!

my home. I had practiced in the lake and had gone on a training ride, but now I had to put it all together.

The swim took me one hour and 18 minutes, the bike ride two hours and 18 minutes, and the run one hour and 49 minutes. With the addition of transition time, my total was 5 hours, 37 minutes. Whew!

True, I was the last to finish; but the clock was still going, and my husband and the race director, plus a few volunteers, cheered me on. I had a great sense of accomplishment!

In the fall, I finished six more running events, including a destination 5K in Seattle and a 5K aboard a Caribbean cruise in December. It was so much fun!

2012

This year, I completed my first half marathon. It was memorable because I did it with my husband, son and daughter-in-law in Seattle. Although I was the last of the group to finish, it was a great sense of accomplishment to run 13.1 miles. This was also Richard's first half marathon.

During the summer, I completed three sprint triathlons and one Olympic distance, again in Maple Grove, Minnesota. Since I had not trained for this distance, my total time was slower than 2011, at just over six hours.

2013

In 2013, I did the most events to date—nineteen! I did something every month, including my second destination triathlon in Key West, Florida. How invigorating to swim in the ocean and then bike and run in the Florida sunshine! This is now one of my favorites.

In May of 2013, I was honored to be awarded Fitness Person of the Year at the St. Paul YWCA and later presented with an 8x10 photo commemorating my achievement. It made my heart sing to see what I had accomplished so far and how it was acknowledged publicly.

I also tried a new distance, a 10-mile run. This is a shorter event during

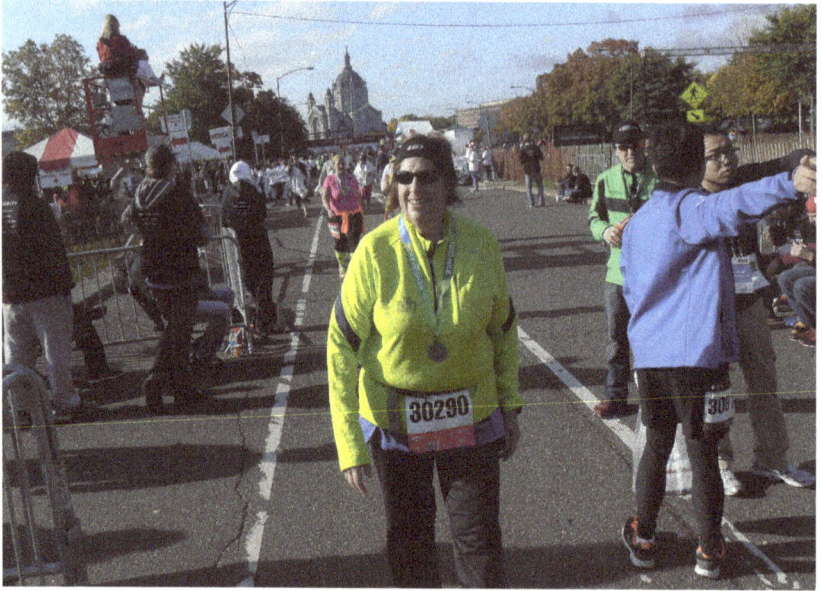

Twin Cities 10 Mile in 2013

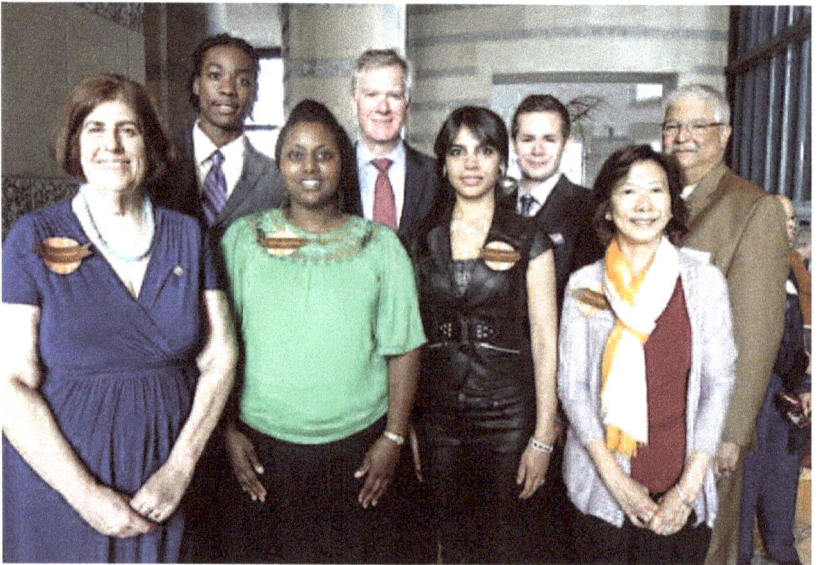

One of four YWCA Sweet Success award winners in 2013

the famous Twin Cities Marathon. The tagline for it is "A Shortcut to the Capitol" since it starts in Minneapolis and cuts out over 16 miles by going directly to St. Paul and running along famed Summit Avenue to cheers of encouragement.

Our winter destination event was in Palm Springs, California where Richard ran a half marathon and I ran a 5K. We also had fun on a bike tour of Palm Springs that highlighted famous houses. We earned a "brick" for doing both events in the same week. (A brick is two events back to back. The Palm Springs people actually gave each of us a brick with a plaque on it.)

This year, I also participated in three summer sprint triathlons and two duathlons, ending the year with a Christmas 5K in Minnesota.

2014

I finished 20 events in 2014, the most in any year, with a mixture of road races and triathlons. This year, our winter destination event was in Augusta, Georgia where I ran a 10K and Richard finished a half marathon. Doing destination events has been a fun February activity for several years. When you live in Minnesota, it's especially enjoyable to go somewhere warm in winter and do a running event.

Richard and I also participated in two duathlons and three triathlons, as well as several 5Ks and 10Ks. It was really fun for us to do our own distances for running races as Richard is great at half marathons and a 10K run was still a challenge for me.

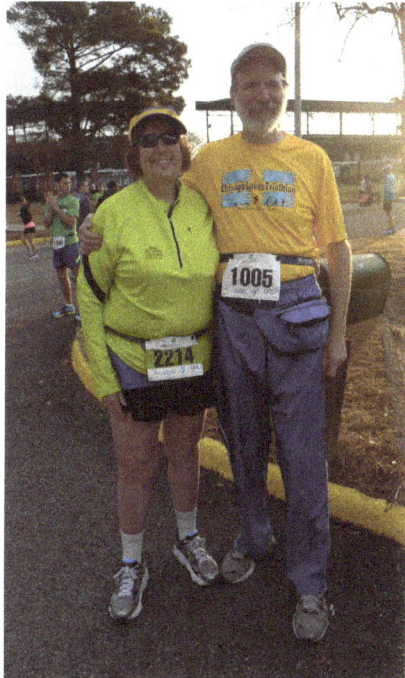

2014 Augusta, Georgia winter event

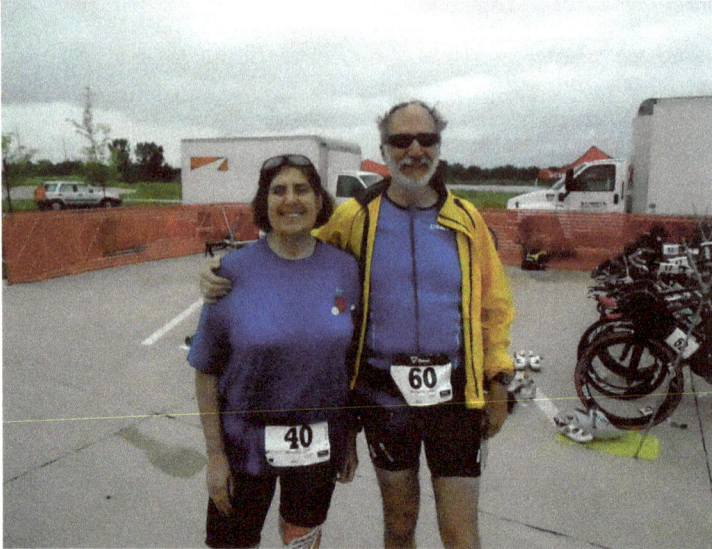

2014 Iowa Duathlon Picture

2015

This year was split into two parts, before and after my March surgery. In January, I did a 10K (Richard, a half marathon) and then in March, we did a 5K together. We skipped our usual February destination event in 2015 because of my surgery.

Surgery

I had surgery to remove the excess skin that was left after my weight loss of over 160 pounds. I needed to be near goal weight so the surgery would be the most effective. It was painful, but I loved that my body now matched how I felt. I had a flat stomach and no more fat pockets on my thighs. I now looked good and felt confident in a swimsuit, and you can really see the difference in these before and after photos.

Unfortunately, I really had trouble slowing down after the surgery to let the healing take place. I exercised too much and finally had to be very careful not to walk more than a few minutes at a time. I kept up my weekly consultations with Keith, and it helped that someone still considered me an athlete.

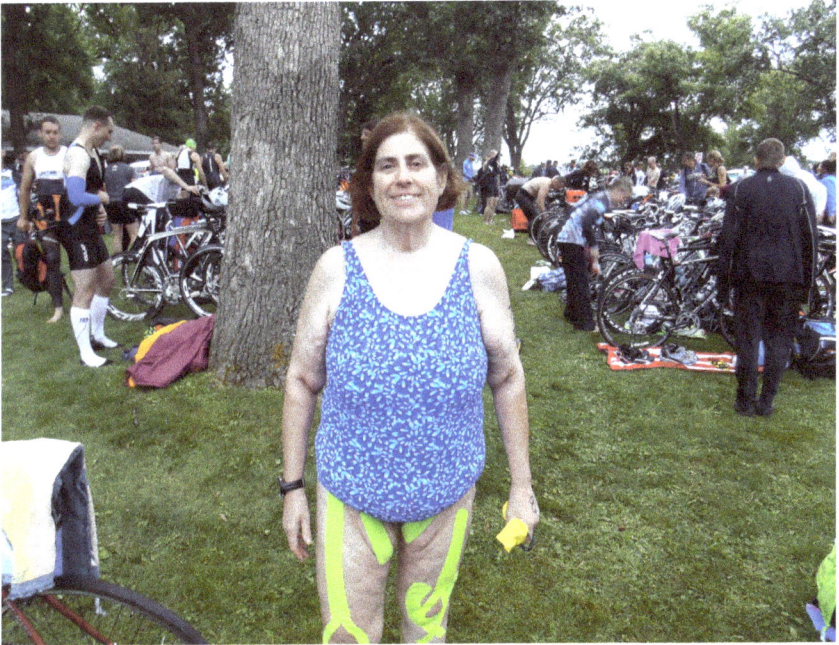

Before Surgery

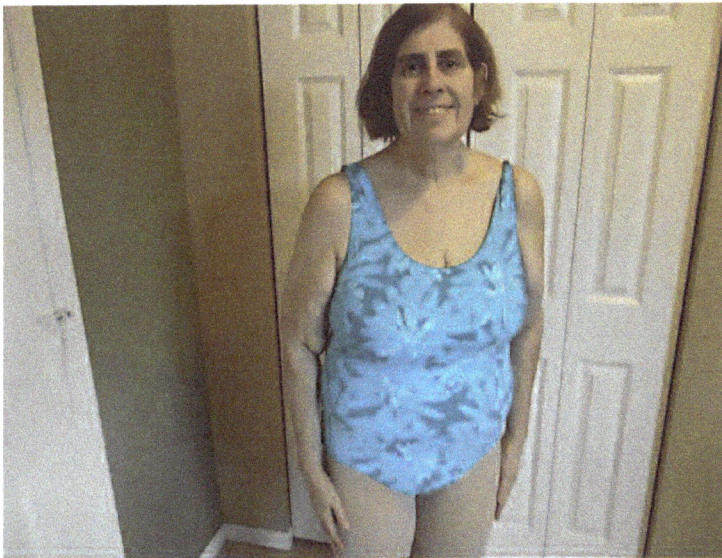

After Surgery

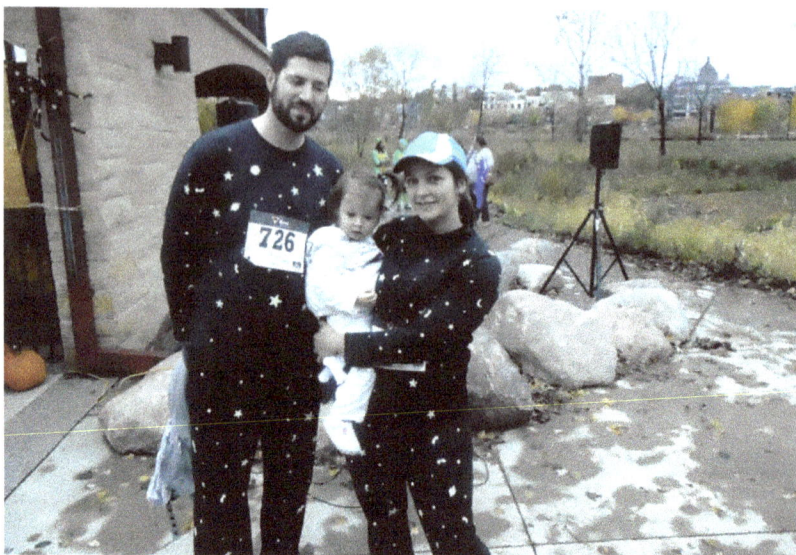

Boo Run Run family support: Noah, Brianna and Evelyn

Beginning in June, I ran a 5K and a 10K each month until finally, in September, I finished a sprint triathlon.

Again, I did the Twin Cities 10 Mile and the Seattle Half Marathon, proudly finishing that event 24 minutes faster than in 2012.

In October 2015, we also did our first three-generation family event, the Boo Run Run 5K.

Richard and I were joined by Noah, Brianna and Evelyn for a 5K in St. Paul. Noah ran with Evelyn in a backpack child carrier. It was not Noah's best time but was a fabulous family event!

I planned to end the year with the Key West Triathlon, but the weather was cloudy and cold. I chickened out of doing the entire event. Instead, Richard and I did it as a relay. He swam. I biked, and then he ran. We finished and had fun!

2016

2016 started out with the usual mix of running events in the winter and spring. One fun destination event was a 10K in Chicago while visiting

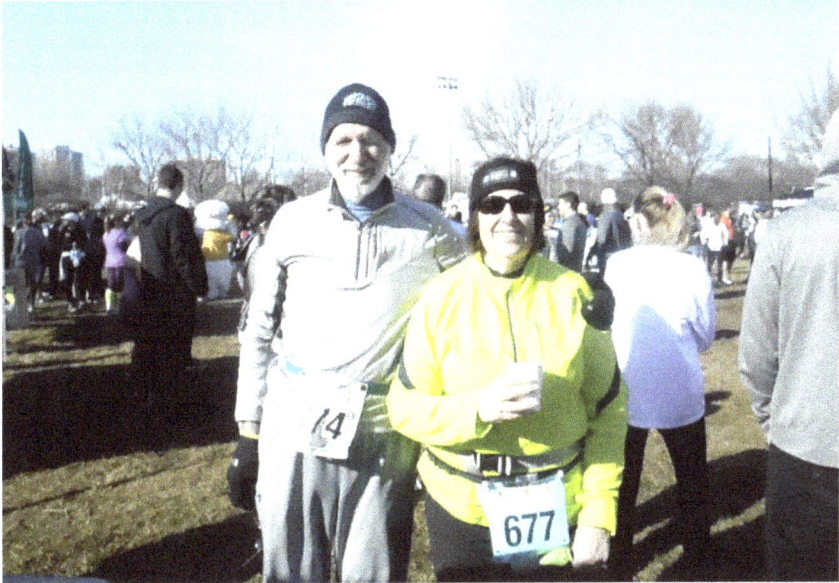

Mardi Gras 10K in Chicago

friends. We found it really enjoyable to combine traveling with athletic events.

This was the year that I could really focus on triathlons since I had now fully recovered from the surgery. I trained for Olympic distance, started seven events and finished six.

My First DNF (Did Not Finish)

My first scheduled triathlon of 2016 was for early June but got started late because of several thunderstorms. We decided not to participate because our bikes and bike shoes were soaked, and it was still cold and rainy.

Therefore, I was emotionally and physically ready for the first triathlon of the year in a lovely venue near the Twin Cities: Annandale. It is called the Heart of the Lakes Triathlon because it circles several area lakes.

The swim in Pleasant Lake was a half mile, and I finished it in 47 minutes. There is a soft cutoff of two hours for the bike and swim, so I knew I had to push myself on the 21-mile bike ride. About 45 minutes into the ride, I hit a rumble strip along the side of the road and fell, bending my bike frame. Someone saw me and stayed with me until an SAG (Support and Gear) vehicle picked me up. I was not badly injured, just my pride. This was my first DNF in 151 events!

I finished the year participating in six more triathlons. Although I had sometimes registered for the Olympic distance, I occasionally changed it to sprint. Each time, I placed first or second in my age group, and by the end of the season, I received three invitations to the USA Triathlon (USAT) National Age Group Olympic Distance event to be held in August of 2017.

For my final triathlon of the year, in Key West, I finished the Olympic distance in 4:49:32—nearly one hour faster than in 2012. I was getting older and better!

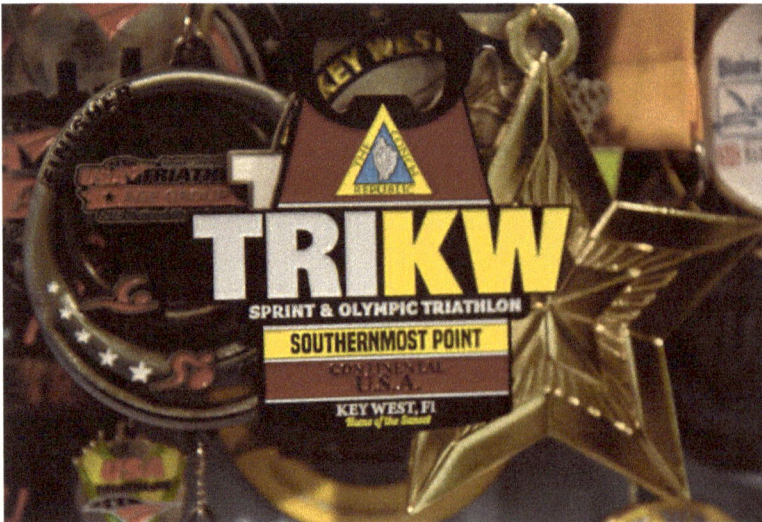

2016 Key West Tri

2017

One of my goals for 2017 was to work on performance at Olympic triathlons. I had attended the National Sprint Race in 2016, in which anyone can participate. Because of my placing first or second in several USAT-sanctioned races, I had now received three invitations to the Olympic Distance event for 2017.

My training changed in significant ways since my goal was not to be a participant but to become a competitive athlete. For 2017, my training included the following:

1. I would only participate in Olympic distance events. Keith's goal for me was 13 and I agreed.

2. I would start my new periodization in February, and it would be variable for the entire 26 weeks.

3. I would need to train with him in the Dominican Republic three times (March, May and July).

4. Another goal was to lose an additional 20 pounds, so I could do the training necessary to become more competitive.

Not all went according to plan. Although I started seven triathlons, I only completed two. It was a new experience to not finish events. Some of the factors that kept me from completing them were bad weather, needing to swim in a wetsuit and mechanical problems with my bike.

Also, when I trained in March, Keith noticed I had begun to de-train. Because of stress in my personal life, I was not making progress. Keith took immediate corrective action, including adding another training session with him in the Dominican Republic in April, upping the weekly consultations to twice a week, and changing my periodization plan by adding more strength training minutes and eliminating the higher intensity minutes. That's what I call *focus!*

Sometimes you just need more support! It's not a failure, but a realization, that life is distracting you in ways you hadn't noticed or comprehended. This is also why I needed that formal support team!

2017 Triathlons

March in Palm Springs, California was my first destination triathlon of the year, and it required a wetsuit. I learned that the use of wetsuits is determined

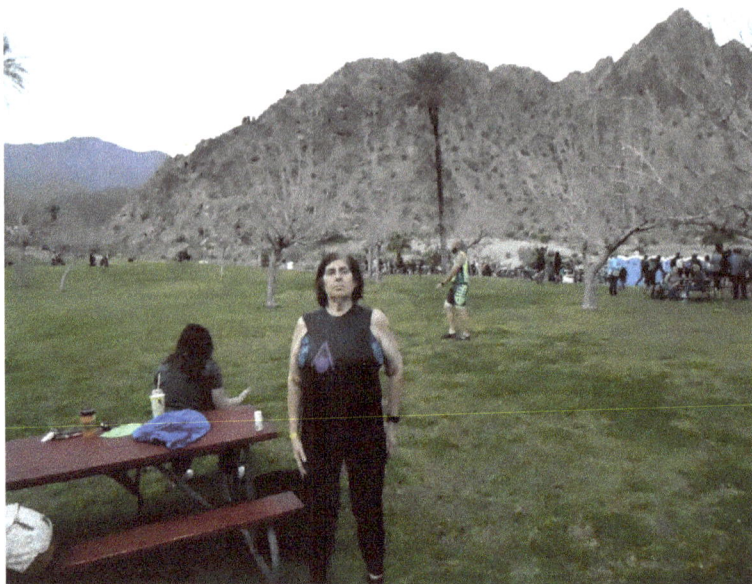

My first wetsuit event in Palm Springs

by the lake temperature. USA Triathlon says that if the water temperature is below 78 degrees, wetsuits are legal. From 78.1 to 83.9 degrees, they may be worn, but a participant is not eligible for an award. For water temperatures at 84 or above, wetsuits are not allowed because of safety reasons (one would overheat).

I practiced the day before the event in a wetsuit for the first time. On the day of the event, I was able to complete the swim in 1 hour, 15 minutes, which is slow. Then, I was able to get out of the wetsuit and start on the bike leg of the event, but because I was so far behind the other riders and some of the bike course was not well marked, I got lost and came back in after 1 hour, 13 minutes.

From this experience, I learned that I needed to drive the bike route before an event since it is always my responsibility to know the route. Thus, the first Olympic of the year was a DNF (Did Not Finish). June had three triathlons scheduled because Keith wanted me to experience overload. I finished the first one in Green Bay, Wisconsin although I was last. The main reason for that was that the half-mile swim was in a man-made lake that allowed for part of the course to be run in the water because it was so shallow. My total time was 4 hours, 24 minutes, and I finished first in my age group.

The second triathlon was west of St. Paul in a beautiful lake. This was the Liberty Triathlon. Unfortunately, it was an extremely windy day and, after nearly one hour in the water, I was pulled from the lake. The race director makes this determination if it is a safety issue for the swimmer. I really felt badly until I learned the following week that 14 people had been pulled from the water.

I was really ready for the third triathlon of the month in nearby Rochester, Minnesota. It was a beautiful day, and the lake in an old quarry was calm. I finished the swim in 1 hour, 27 minutes and got on my bike. I got to the turnaround and, on the way back, was biking into a headwind. Then, bad luck struck at Mile 18, and my bike tire went flat. There was no support available, so I had to end the race.

July's first race was the Timberman Triathlon held at a lovely resort in northern Minnesota. Luckily, the water was warm, so I didn't need to worry about a wetsuit. I spoke to the race director to find out if there was a time limit, and he said no. I drove the route with Richard and was prepared for the rolling hills of the course. There were two loops, one shorter than the other. I started off with the swim and finished in 1 hour, 27 minutes. I got through Loop One and was ready for Loop Two when the race director pulled me from the race. It turns out there was a time limit as the volunteers needed to vacate the course after 11:30 AM.

The director said I could run a shorter version of 1.5 miles. Therefore, I finished a race although not at an Olympic distance. (I was disappointed because I would have been second in my age group and received a prize.)

By this point, I was really discouraged. I had never had so many DNFs. I began dreading the triathlons instead of enjoying them. During my July training trip, Keith explained the following to me:

1.   My goal was to be competitive, not just to finish an event. My success

should be measured by how consistently I do my training. In fact, I had not continued to de-train but had made enough progress that he added more challenging strength routines and added back more high intensity aerobic minutes. That was encouraging to hear.

2. I do not need to train to finish sprint distances, and in fact, I am better suited for the endurance aspect of the Olympic distance.

3. I need to keep focusing on my weight loss goals. One way to accomplish this will be to stabilize my training and eating times to the same schedule for the day of the week.

Not meeting my goals was difficult for me. I had been really proud of having only one DNF after 160 events from 2007–2016. However, I had to remember that 2017 had begun a new phase where I was working toward becoming a competitive athlete, not merely a participant in events.

My sixth race was the Turtleman on July 29th at Turtle Lake near St. Paul. Again, I finished the swim, this time in 1 hour, 47 minutes. I started the bike route and did one loop, but because it was a hot day and I was tired from the long swim time, I chose not to finish.

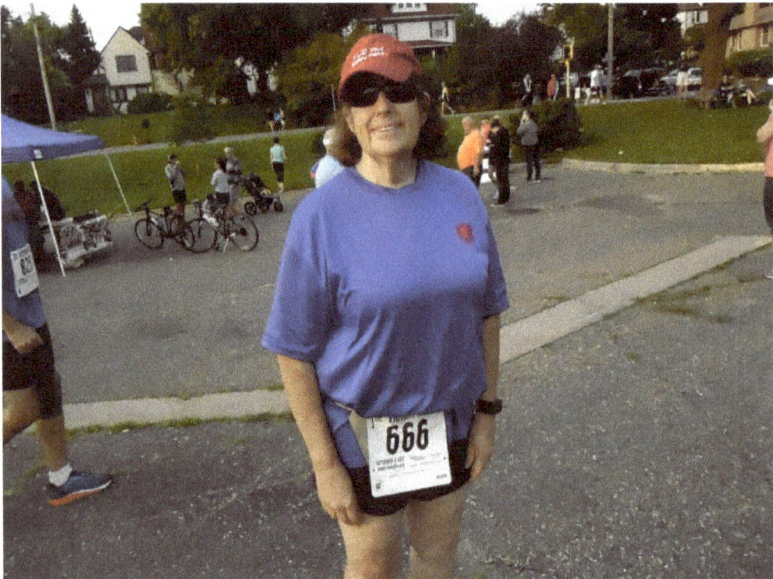

Monster Dash 10 Mile

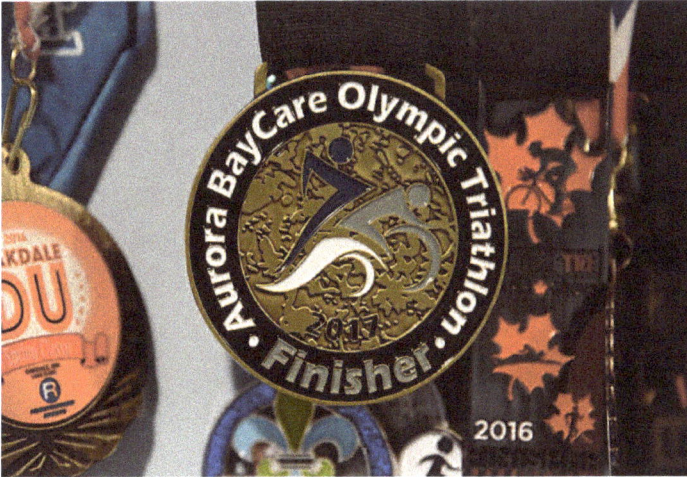

Finisher Medal from the Aurora BayCare Olympic Triathlon

Nationals

Then, on August 13, I was ready for the USA Triathlon Age Group Nationals in Omaha, Nebraska. I finished! My total time was 5 hours, 55 minutes. Because I placed 32 out of 32 participants in my age group, I will not participate in the ITU World Age group race in Australia in 2018.

Post National

After the Omaha event, I changed my training to the post-season phase which lasted six weeks. I trained with Keith one last time in September and started my off-season phase. I was now focusing on strength training, and my aerobics minutes were in the three lowest ranges.

My events in these two phases had also changed. For my September birthday treat, Richard and I ran a 10K, the Victory 10K in Minneapolis. During October, I participated in two 10-mile races in St. Paul.

Not meeting all my goals was difficult indeed, but every journey has its ups and downs. The important lessons I've learned from 2017 are:

1. Not all goals can be accomplished, especially when you are challenging yourself.
2. A competitive athlete needs a regular schedule in as many areas

as possible. This includes nutrition, the times you train and the contents of that training.

3. DNFs are not failures. How you do during an event is not as important as the training to get there and the lessons learned.

I was really looking forward to finishing the year in Key West, Florida. It is my favorite triathlon—swimming, biking and running in the Florida sunshine in December. The weather was fantastic from Tuesday to Friday. Then, Friday night, the weather changed, and a heavy thunderstorm came through. First, the swim portion was cancelled, then the entire triathlon. Luckily, our registration was forwarded to 2018. December 1, 2018 is the date!

2018

This year got off to a great start with training in the Dominican Republic with Keith during the second week of January. I was happy to know that he saw improvement since our September training. As I was still in the off season, we planned to focus this next cycle on strength training and weight training. I will work out five days a week, focusing on aerobics and a strength routine and take two days off.

My event goals are also very different for this year. My periodization will begin in June, and I will do two Olympic lengths in August and December. I can do as many sprint triathlons as I want and any road races. My plans are to do a road race each month through May and a sprint triathlon in June, July and August.

I am looking forward to a great 2018!

My Training Journey

My fitness journey of events was coordinated and supported by my training journey. Depending on the season, level of progress or stage of year, my training changed under Keith's direction.

There are two basic components of each regimen—aerobics and strength—with flexibility being the foundation for all training plans. To recount each routine would not be helpful or instructive, but there are lessons I have learned about training that need to be considered.

1. Listen to your trainer.

When I was a new mother, I once had a criticism about my pediatrician. My mother listened to me recount the story and replied that when you hire a professional you either listen and follow their advice or find a new one. The same is true of a trainer. Keith always says, "Don't be creative. Do what I instruct you." I could not have made this progress without listening to him. If you are not willing to listen, you either need another trainer or a different attitude.

2. Strength training needs to be progressive.

As I lost weight and gained strength and ability, my strength training changed. From fitness bands and later fitness cuffs, I progressed to dumbbells and barbells. The specifics will depend on what you are trying to accomplish and must be supervised by a qualified trainer. If I just keep doing the same exercises month after month, I will not make progress in achieving my goals. In fact, becoming too efficient is not generally a helpful goal if I do not strive to progressively challenge myself other areas of my training.

3. Being open to trying new things.

I grew up in the 1950s before Title IX and before being healthy was a goal. Because of being overweight and experiencing the effects of polio, I wasn't good at most sports or physical activities. My nieces can't believe that girls (we didn't become women until college) were sometimes taught to let boys win because of their fragile egos. Where I grew up, it was acceptable to be smart, but not smart and fit.

Therefore, I had a lot of negative attitudes to overcome. One was that any new activity was going to be hard. Another was that I wasn't going to be good at it, so it scared me. Wrong perspective! To succeed in any fitness journey, I need to be open to new experiences. If I'm not perfect the first time, so what? That is why I'm training. I'm learning to use my body in new ways.

I often remind myself to think about what I can do, not what I can't. (See more in Chapter 5, "Attitude and Perspective.")

Sometimes I would ask Keith about a certain exercise and ask if I could do that. Later, when I had made the appropriate progress, it was added to my regimen.

Now I have the pride of accomplishment when I can discuss my routine with colleagues 20 years younger and find I am doing the same exercises they do!

4. Understanding my training cycle.

I do not do the same strength routines all year. Besides focusing on improvement, they are also dependent on where I am in my training cycle. Even if I am not training for events, I learned the value of having training cycles all year round. In 2016, I had several eight-week cycles before and after my six-month periodization.

My Nutrition Journey

I do not call this a "diet journey" because I believe the word "diet" has too many negative and unrealistic connotations. Every January, the ads start in magazines and on TV that imply that, with little effort and lots of money, you can become thin. Bariatric surgery for the morbidly obese has its own series! In this section, I will again chronicle what I have learned. This is the part of the journey that has been the most difficult as I keep learning more about nutrition. I am not yet at my weight goal but, with the resources I have, I keep trying.

Step 1: Just eat less.

Getting active helped me lose weight, but I still needed to change my eating habits. The first actions I took were to make changes by just eating less of the unhealthy foods that had become commonplace in my daily routine. I used to love hash browns, but the first change that Keith asked of me was to eat half as much of them. Now, I never order them and even the taste is no longer appetizing. So, if there is a food you love that is not the healthiest, you can start by eating less.

Step 2: Sometimes cold turkey is best.
Keith challenged me to stop eating fast food. Most of the fast-food meals are high in fat and sodium. Even "healthy" salads do not always use nutritious greens. So, before my first grandchild was born, I stopped eating fast foods. That was October of 2007.

Step 3: Make modifications.
I loved mochas, chocolate, coffee, Espresso and whipped cream. What's not to love? I really don't want to live in a world without chocolate, but even a mocha can be modified to be healthier. I order a small with skim, less chocolate and no whip, and I still have a delicious treat.

Step 4: Get professional help.
There are both dieticians and nutritionists who can help, and sometimes health insurance will cover the cost. I have worked through the years with several different programs and professionals. There are also helpful computer programs and apps for smartphones. The most important lesson I learned is that it is important to log what I eat.

In the fall of 2007, I started my nutritional counseling with Keith. He created a nutrition and dietary accountability and proactive programming dietary intake log we used for several years to help me lose weight by proactively controlling my meals. We used this tool as a part of our weekly coaching sessions to help me prepare for events. It has been extremely challenging for me, but it is what works more than any other program I have used. Again, having a support team helps.

Step 5: Log food intake.

If I want to make progress, I know I need to track my food, the amounts, when I eat and, at a minimum, the calories, fat, protein and carbohydrates. Everyone's nutritional needs are different, so it is beyond the scope of this book to make specific recommendations. Just be certain that there is science behind the chosen plan or program. I want to live in the real world where I travel, go out to eat and meet with friends over food. I can do that, make healthy choices and enjoy myself.

I also learned the importance of drinking water. My goal was to drink one ounce of water daily for every pound of weight.

Step 6: Get information about food.

The internet is a great resource for information. Here are some ideas for resources that I have used:

A. **Google it.** Search for a food by "nutritional value in [*name of food*]." This is great for unusual or multi-ingredient foods.

B. **Find nutritional data** on websites nutritiondata.self.com or calorieking.com.

C. **My Fitness Pal.** The one caveat here is that some information is supplied by users, so it may not be completely accurate.

D. **Lose It!** This app is similar to My Fitness Pal with free and paid plans.

E. **Websites for chain restaurants.** This is handy when traveling. Most major chains have fit or healthy menus. Be aware! Low calories may or may not be healthy for you. I am trying to limit fat and even an omelet with egg whites can have more fat than you realize. Another caveat about chain restaurant meals is that steamed is better than grilled. Grilling adds fat.

F. **CSPI.Net** (Center for Science and Public Interest). Their website nutrition.com is not privately funded. It is like consumer reports for nutrition. In Keith's opinion this is THE MOST important nutrition resource there is today.

G. **USDA** (US Department of Agriculture). The USDA has the Super-tracker and choosemyplate.gov weekly digest. Keith says this is one of the best resources you can find, with no vested interests and all publicly funded.

Shopping for groceries can be fun! With the abundance of fresh fruit and vegetables and readily available entrée choices, I can create eye-appealing, delicious meals without sacrificing nutritional value. I prepare a carefully considered shopping list and mainly shop the perimeter of the grocery store since that's where the whole foods reside. The inner aisles are primarily dedicated to pre-packaged convenience and processed foods. However, this is where I also find spices, oils and other simple ingredients for cooking basics.

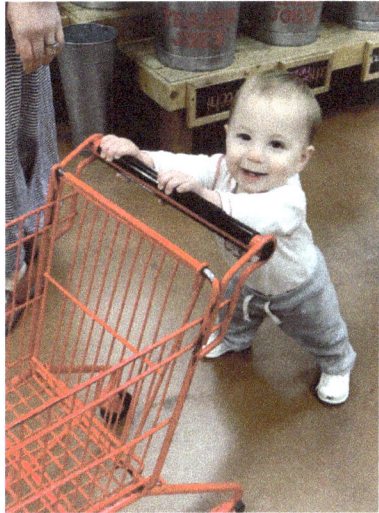

Grandson Asher—Nutritional shopper in training

Step 7: Prepare weekly meal plans.

Another tool that Keith trained me on was to proactively plan my meals on a weekly basis. Keith is always telling me I know exactly how many minutes I will exercise every day for months, so why not know what I will eat for at least one week! The concept is that each day of the week I know what I'm going to eat at each meal. The goal is to keep my calories and nutrients the same each day. If I go out, I can plan that ahead of time also. See Step 4: Get professional help. When I travel, I know what foods to bring or buy if there is a refrigerator in the room. Also, I know what portions to order in a restaurant.

Since I am serious about my fitness and meal choices, meal planning really helps me with my weight loss goals. The same plan would be helpful if I had a medical condition that required food modifications. If I needed to limit sodium, for example, I could read food labels to find out which foods are better and which to avoid. I believe many restaurants are now using less salt since so many people need to limit sodium, but I don't make assumptions. I will ask if the salt can be adjusted.

Step 8: It all takes time.

Learning a healthy relationship with food was difficult and took a lot of effort and emotional growth for me. It takes time. Although I am not yet at my goal weight, I have not gained weight. Sometimes not making progress is frustrating, but I do not consider this a failure.

I also found new ways to treat myself that didn't involve food. Some ideas were to go to a movie with a friend, go to a play or visit an art museum. It was essential for me to celebrate achievements and successes without food.

SECTION TWO

LESSONS LEARNED

Chapter 2

The Importance of Balance

I realize no one can ever be completely in balance. Throughout my day, week, month and year, there are few times when I am completely balanced. I've learned that the goal here is to work toward balance. At the end of the day, I'm happy that I can say that most of the time I am balanced.

There are many representations of balance (just Google Balance—Images), and for me, the most apt one is a wheel. For a wheel or a life to move forward the entire whole needs to be in balance. I define a complete life balance as SEMPS:

S	Social
E	Emotional
M	Mental
P	Physical
S	Spiritual

I learned these from my first mentor, Marq Stankowski, who saw something in a very young and inexperienced college student when he gave me responsibilities for documenting a summer program he had directed.

SEMPS

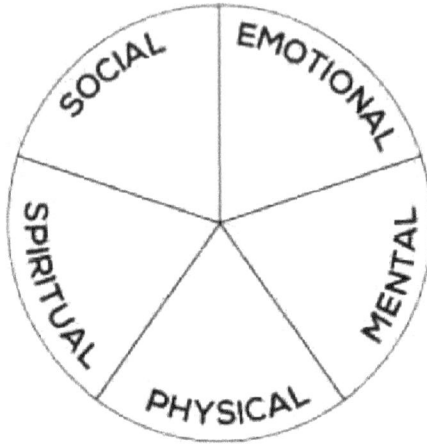

So how do these components help with balance? One needs to have some of each—not too much and not too little—to be at peace.

Social—This is your relationship with friends and family. We all know social butterflies who are always going to events, and other people who are more solitary, going it alone. When you are socially in balance, you have friends and family that you enjoy. You have activities that you share. As you begin a fitness journey, your social relationships may change. You may have less time to hang out, and you may make new friends that share your new interests.

Emotional—This is your inner life, what you see in the mirror in the morning. An emotionally healthy person is self-aware, not self-absorbed. Being in balance emotionally means you are integrated and you see yourself as others see you. You know yourself and understand your strengths and weaknesses. Being in balance emotionally will help you make progress on your fitness journey.

Mental—This is your intellect and intelligence. Keith always has said he likes to train smart people because they know how to learn. You need to be a learner if you are going to be successful on a fitness journey. You may need to take classes or get a trainer. It will help if you enjoy learning. The more you learn about your body and how it operates, the better for you and your progress.

Physical—This was the part of my life that was not in balance before I began my fitness journey. The Greeks talked of a sound mind in a sound body. I am proud of my body now and proud of my accomplishments.

Spiritual—This is the part of your life that is deeply personal. For some, it is a connection with an established religion, for others it is more a quest for spirituality. Some find it in native religions or meditation. Finding expression in this aspect of life helps round out individual qualities and a sense of balance.

So how do we achieve Balance? By being aware of these aspects in our lives and finding ways to nurture and enhance them. Balance will look differently for each of us. You will know when you are in that state, and you will be better for it.

Chapter 3

A Support Team

Importance of a Support Team

Early in my training with Keith, I spoke very dispiritedly to him that it was taking three people to keep me going that winter: Keith, Jeanne Heald, my life coach, and Dave Peterson, my massage therapist. Keith answered, "Because you are smart." I then realized that having a formal support team is smart. I have expanded the concept to business presentations for small- to medium-sized businesses or SMEs as well with great success.

Formal Support Team

No person is an island. In my experience, the support of professionals, family and friends in reaching my fitness goals cannot be overstated. Some of the people that I count on now or have used on my fitness journey include a primary care physician, medical specialists for my particular health issues, a fitness trainer, a psychologist, a dietician or nutritionist, kinesio taping specialist, manual therapist, and a massage therapist.

My Support Team Members:

1. **An ACSM-certified personal trainer** (trained to work with a person like me)

For my fitness journey, this is an essential member of my team. I could not have accomplished what I have without Keith Gosline, founder of Personal Fitness Systems and owner of Gosline-MAPP, SRL in Santo Domingo, Dominican Republic.

It may cost more and take more time to find the right trainer, but it is an essential component to learning safe and effective routines.

It is also important that my primary physician approved me for exercises.

2. **Psychologist**

Dr. Emily Fields has been an important member of my formal support team. Since 2006, I have needed help understanding the changes I have made and how they have impacted relationships with both family and business clients. Knowing I needed this help, I was not afraid to seek assistance.

3. **Dietician/Nutritionist**

I knew that at some point in my fitness journey, I would need some professional help in managing my diet. There are many plans out there, and it is beyond the scope of this book to evaluate these plans. I found it helpful to meet with a dietician and nutritionist to discuss my goals and hear their assessment and advice. Some health clinics have a professional on staff.

Here are some factors I considered important:
   A. A person with credentials from a national organization.
   B. A person (sports nutritionist) who understands the nutritional needs of athletes.
   C. A plan that can be maintained. (Remember: *No Quick Fixes!*)
   D. A plan that emphasizes real food and that is flexible enough for my lifestyle.

4. Physician or Other Medical Professional

I recognized the need for a medical professional who would support my journey. Keith insisted that I have physician approval before I could begin, and my doctor was supportive and has been proud of my achievements. Some medicines might help; but, again, I didn't feel that was a permanent solution for me (although I did use an appetite suppressant for about six months).

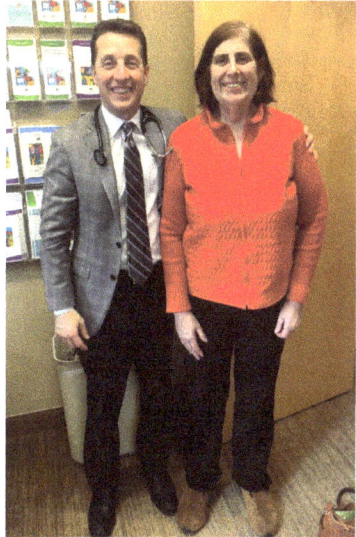

My cardiologist, Dr. Katsiyiannis, and me

My primary physician, Dr. John Beecher, has been pleased with my fitness journey. In the beginning, I weighed in with him every 3–4 months, but now I only see him once a year for my annual physical.

In addition, my cardiologist, Dr. Katsiyiannis, has been a great source of encouragement. I started with annual visits and now only need to see him every two years. At my last visit, he asked if his nurse could take a picture of us to show his other patients. What an honor—and another type of celebration. Who doesn't want to be a model patient for a heart doctor?

5. Massage Therapist

Ann Short is my Minnesota massage therapist. She and Keith were colleagues in the past, so Keith knew that she would provide the services I needed once Keith had moved to the Dominican Republic. At each visit, I get a massage, and, before some events, I get a massage that is targeted for my immediate needs.

Informal Support Team

My informal support team includes the people in my personal life who will help me. They are members of my family, neighbors, friends, business colleagues, co-workers and trusted members of my professional groups and business organizations. As I progress, these people notice the changes. As I reach barriers, these are the people I trust and can turn to for help.

Some other members of my informal support team have been my fellow triathletes and race participants. I learned this during my first race when one of the runners came back to run with me to the finish line. Another example was when the fellow swimmers cheered me on as I finished the indoor swim in Alexandria. Here is that picture:

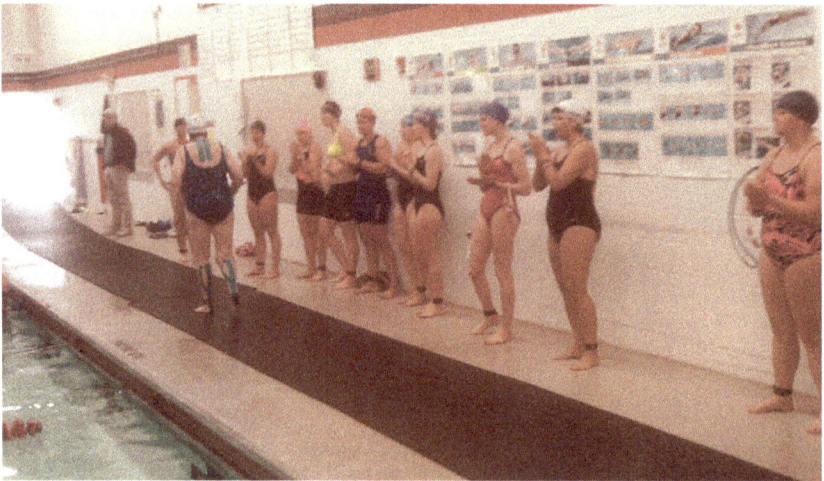

Alexandria Triathlon

In my experience, triathletes are supportive of each other. Even the elite athletes have acknowledged my efforts with a High Five or a "Good going!"

Another informal support team member has been Gary Westlund of Charities Challenge. His nonprofit organization sponsors 5K races for holidays or challenges such as obesity or diabetes. During the Twin Cities Marathon, he mans a booth and runs out to take my picture as I run the ten mile.

Here are some pictures from his events:

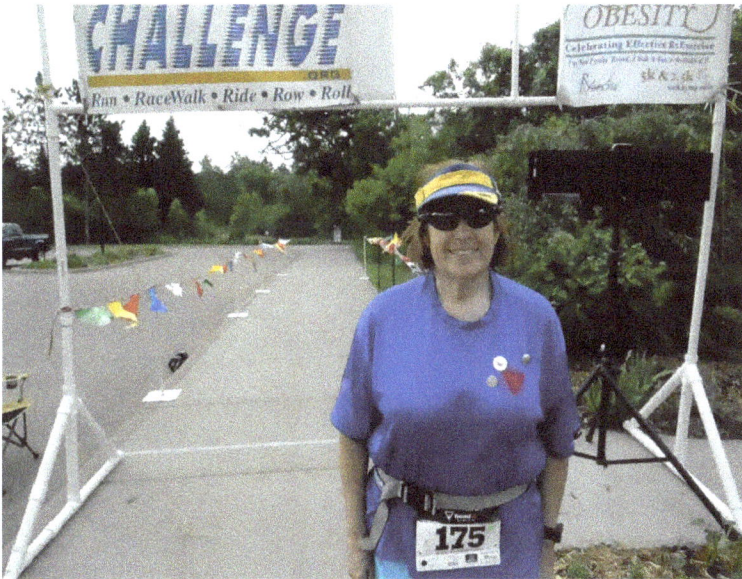

June 2015 Charities Challenge Obesity Event,
Bunker Hills Park, Andover, MN

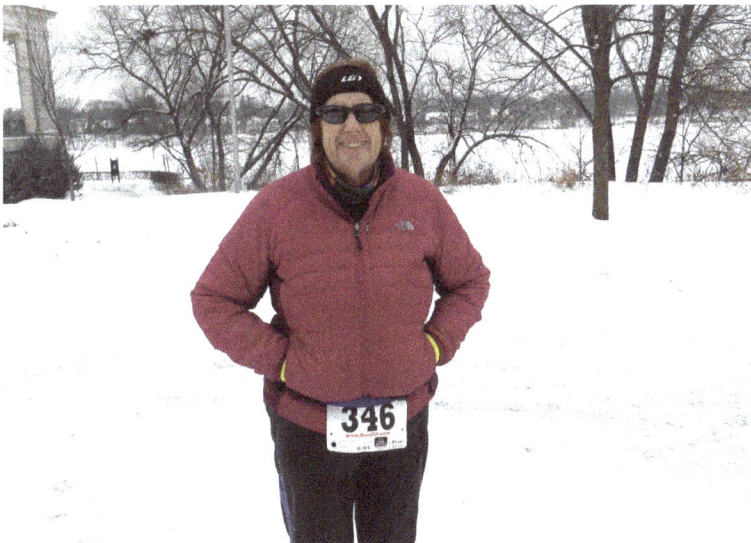

December 25, 2015 Charities Challenge Joyful 5K Event,
Como Park, St. Paul, MN

My family has always been an important part of my informal support team. This has included my siblings, Charlie, Varda and Elinor, who always want to hear about my latest race. My mother has always been interested in hearing about my races and is so proud of me. Although she cannot be at my events in person anymore, she is eager to hear about them. She was also impressed to see the new Specialized bike that I recently purchased.

Of particular help is Richard Weil, my husband of 43 years. In the first few years of my fitness journey, he came to every event to cheer me on. In fact, the first event he did not attend was a 5K I did in Las Vegas in October 2007 while vacationing with our younger son.

Later, Richard started joining in on events because, as he said, he got tired of waiting around for me to finish. He found out that he is a runner and finished half marathons in the 2-hour, 30-minute range. He even trained with Keith and successfully completed his first marathon, the Twin Cities, in 2014.

Members of BNI (Business Network International), a networking and referral organization, have always been part of my informal team. They have been interested in my accomplishments and events. I've also helped others begin their fitness journeys, and we've added outdoor activities to some of our summer events.

Some members of my support team have been able to support me even better when I have explained the process, training, education and support and have answered their questions. For example, I have asked my mother to have fresh fruit at Thanksgiving. Another way my family has been able to promote my weight loss is to avoid bringing sweets into the house. When my husband buys the Halloween candy, I ask him to put it away and out of my sight. I don't want to be tempted.

Exercise Facilities

Even though a fitness facility is not a support person for my team, it does play an important role in supporting my efforts and fitness success. When I was new to training, I thought all gyms and facilities are about the same, but clearly, they are not. Some places are just pickup places for young people. Being middle aged and overweight, I did not feel comfortable in such places.

Here's what I learned about exercise facilities and how I have chosen those that have served me well:

1. Location

If it is convenient to get to, with easy parking, I am more likely to use it. The location should be near my work and/or home so getting there can be a part of my new routine.

2. Cost

Different places have different policies. It is important to me to review the contracts ahead of time. Often health insurance will cover a joiner fee or part of my monthly membership. I am not going to be coerced into a contract until I have used the facility at times that are convenient for me.

In my experience, good values can be found at city-operated centers and those run by YWCA or YMCA. Both are open to all sexes. Private chains may be more expensive, but when I travel, it may be worth the higher price to have facilities I know in remote locations.

3. Clientele

I prefer to try out a class or two to see who is attending. I am more comfortable if some class members are more similar to me in age, gender and ability. Occasionally, I have attended a step class with a friend, but I wasn't entirely comfortable because I usually could not keep up with the younger women. On the other hand, I have had a great deal of enjoyment with indoor cycling classes and fitness yoga.

My Polio Story

I had polio as a baby in the summer of 1951. This was before the Salk vaccine was developed. My parents didn't know it at the time, and it wasn't discovered until I was about seven years old. One indication of the polio was that I never crawled. I just started walking at 10 months. My parents didn't realize that this was a problem. They just thought I was precocious! (I was their first!) After visiting different orthopedic specialists, it was decided that I needed two operations.

The first was the summer of 1959, the summer before I started 4th grade. Both feet were operated on, including fusing bones in my left foot. Then, my feet were stretched into casts at an angle, so the shorter ligaments would lengthen.

Fourth grade was significant because that was the year we had a separate physical education class. I didn't do well because I was still recovering from surgery. In those days, grades were given if you did or did not reach a certain standard. You were not graded on progress or effort. I realize now that this was a source of my negative attitude toward fitness in general.

The second set of operations was necessary because there was a 1.5-inch difference between my leg lengths. Therefore, metal staples were inserted in my left knee so that it would grow slower and the right leg could catch up. The staples were inserted in 1961 and removed about 18 months later in 1963.

Keith did a lot of research on how polio affected my ability to train and learn. He adjusted his training to include more repetitions of new exercises, and, at times, we would train together several times a week to be certain that I was making appropriate progress, particularly with my strength training.

Chapter 4

Goal Setting

My Principles for Goal Setting

There are some principles that have helped me improve the odds of meeting my goals. I have achieved the most success when the parameters of my goals have been:

1. Measurable.
2. Obtainable.
3. Flexible.

Let me give a few examples:

> When my goal is to work out more, the goal is not measurable.
>
> When my goal is to go instantly from sedentary to a 60-minute step class, the goal not obtainable.
>
> When my goal is to work out every day at exactly 10 AM, the goal is not flexible.

Also, studies have found that if I have a written goal and share it with someone, it is more likely that I will be successful. This is when my informal support team really helps. They can review my goals to be certain they are measurable, obtainable and flexible. They can also help with accountability, which I will discuss in more detail in Chapter 9.

Keith has trained me on another effective tactic which is to set my initial goals at a level slightly less than what I can achieve. An example is the first goal Keith set for me which was three minutes of aerobics a day. This ensured success. Certainly, we could have started at five minutes a day, but three minutes was achievable, measurable and flexible. After that, all I needed was to add one minute per day, each week.

By starting at less than I was capable of, I gained confidence as the minutes per day grew each week. When we worked together, he had me work out for 15 minutes. I gained confidence that I could do it, and by slowly building the number of minutes, I was always successful in meeting my goals. This method is also helping me to reach more goals as I continue my journey.

These principles are used in all areas my life, including my work goals, family financial goals, vacation planning, or whatever part of my life deserves more success.

Here is the step-by-step process I use to achieve my goals:

Step 1: **First, I need to know my weekly goal.** For example, three sessions of strength training for about 30 minutes + 120 minutes of aerobics.

Step 2: **I create a calendar for the week.**

Step 3: **I add my work schedule, including travel time.**

Step 4: **Add family or business commitments.** Perhaps this week is my mother's birthday or my monthly club meeting.

Step 5: **Schedule my workouts.** Allow time for travel to a gym, showering, hair and makeup. It is more helpful to me when I am specific, including minutes and type of activity.

When I don't think I can schedule everything, I get creative. Can I get up 15 minutes earlier and do some calisthenics before work? Can I take a longer lunch hour and fit in a 30-minute walk with a colleague?

Again, this is where my support team is of great help. I gave up some of my more sedentary pursuits, so I would have more time available to work on my health and fitness. What has been important for me is to schedule my workouts with the same mindfulness that I schedule doctor appointments or work hours. I am changing my perspective since I am now an active person who works out on a regular and consistent basis—and it has changed my world!

Chapter 5

Attitude and Perspective

Lessons Learned

1. Focus on what you can do, not what you can't do.

I learned this during my first year of training. Keith suggested I work with him to change my eating habits. I wrote him what I can only describe as a long, tortured email on why I couldn't do it. His reply was to focus on what you can do, not what you can't. This was wisdom I have not forgotten.

This led to me making small changes in my eating habits. Later, I did a couple of months of nutritional counseling with him. I also consulted with a nutritionist and weighed in with my doctor every couple of months.

I have used this lesson several times during my fitness journey. For example, it led to writing this book. My version of this is that it takes just as much time and energy to figure out how not to do something as it does to find a way to do it.

I keep my perspective on the positive, consistently asking myself, "How can I accomplish this goal?" instead of "What are the barriers?" In Chapter 10, I list some of the negative statements that people have said to me and my replies that have helped me focus and succeed.

2. Life is a journey, not a destination.

When I started my fitness journey, I thought there would be an end. I would lose 100 pounds. I would finish an event. I would learn a new sport. But I was wrong. Life is a journey, and it only ends when you stop living.

I have goals that help me move forward, and those goals lead to more goals. When I reach my goal weight, I will have new goals around maintenance and new activities I can try. When I get too old (when I am 90? when I am 100?), there will still be some events I will try. At that point, I will always place in my age group!

This concept became clear to me at the YWCA award ceremony as Fitness Person of the Year in 2013. My good friend and support team member Sean Truman sent me an email that read, "A milestone on your fitness journey." How true that was!

3. Being open to new perspectives.

I learned this during my first year of 5Ks. Each time I finished a 5K, my time was faster until I did a winter race on a very hilly course. I was devastated! Keith had called to see how my race went, and I tearfully told him my time was slower than my last full race. He told me that I can't compare races unless they are on the same course and under the same weather conditions. I tearfully replied, "You never told me that."

He then asked if I had run the last leg up a hill. I replied that yes, I had, and wasn't I supposed to? He told me that many of the half marathon runners had walked it, and so I immediately gained a new perspective. I was better than at least some half marathon runners!

Another new perspective I had to learn was not to compare myself to others. I am very competitive—just ask my son Noah. He'll tell you how I taught him to play checkers without letting him win. He eventually learned how to win legitimately and then had great pride in his wins. I needed to learn that if other participants passed me, I should not compare myself to them. I needed to run the race the way I was trained to run it.

When I ran my first 5K, my goals were to finish and not be last. Keith said to let go of the latter because finishing was the only important thing for me to do. However, there was a mother/daughter team that I kept passing, then they would pass me. I gave a burst at the end and wasn't last!

The perspective is to be a participant in an event. However, years ago I read an article on Active.com that said it is all well and good to be a participant in an event, but sometimes it is fun to win!

I have learned that there are two ways to increase my odds of at least winning my age group:

A. **Participate in smaller events.** If there are fewer participants, I have a greater chance of winning.

B. **Getting older.** Having been born in 1950, I have that wrapped up! In 2016, in five of the six triathlons I participated in, I received either first or second place because I was either the only participant or I was one of two participants in my age group. In fact, I got three separate invitations to the National Olympic Distance Triathlon, sponsored by USAT (USA Triathlon).

Transformation

My fitness journey has not just transformed me from sedentary to athletic but has also transformed me as a person.

One obvious benefit is that I have more confidence. If I can change my body, I can also change other parts of my life. I have more confidence about my abilities and gifts. One example is that I realized that running a business was no longer what I wanted to do, and I had the courage to sell my business in 2015. It was a great decision and I have scaled back from working 30+ hours a month to billing less than 15 hours.

In 2017, I also started a new project writing business plans that is working well. I prepared two business plans, an internal one for a business owner and another for an SBA loan. I look forward to preparing more in 2018.

I am currently working with a colleague to develop workshops for couples who are preparing for retirement. This venture is called Sage Advice for your Retirement Journey.

Thankfully, I gained the courage to learn how to travel alone. If I want to visit my Seattle grandchildren, I can always go there by myself if my husband is not available. I can even travel solo and feel comfortable by myself in another country.

I also became more assertive with my clients. I have transitioned most of them since I sold the business. In the past, I would have apologized or worried that they would be angry or disappointed. Instead, I have calmly told them that I am transitioning away from monthly clients. Each positive response made it easier and easier.

Another way I have been assertive is that I have chosen to continue training with Keith in the Dominican Republic, with weekly online coaching sessions as well.

Training as a Life Focus

When I first started training, I was working full time as a business owner. In those days, I would schedule clients, then my training. As I am transitioning towards retirement, I schedule training first, then clients. In fact, my training schedule does not change now in each cycle. As much as possible, I do my regimens at the same time every day. Training frames my day and week, then I get the rest of my life done.

I have found that I get more accomplished when I am committed to my workouts. At the end of the day, when I email my daily activity log to Keith, it is motivating to know I have done what was prescribed for me that day. As I am transitioning towards retirement, I have also realized that I will be spending much more of my life in the future working out than working!

Even with a full-time job, as a business owner or parent, my fitness journey is a priority and requires focus as well as commitment. In the section on barriers, I share my ideas on how I have been able to overcome them and stay positive.

Chapter 6

Celebration

Jeanne also taught me the importance of celebration. I have used this concept in several ways.

Affirmation Statements

First, I made a list of celebration statements or affirmations. These can be personal or something to say to myself during an event. For example, for swimming, I might say it is a beautiful day for a swim or might compare myself to a dolphin.

For running, I think of going as fast as a roadrunner. "Beep, Beep."

For biking, I don't need an affirmation because riding a bike makes me feel like a kid again.

Keith came up with a new affirmation for me for 2017—and I like it!

Because I can.
Because I like it.
Because it's good for me.

This is one I am also using for 2018. These three phrases can be used in many ways, such as:

a) When starting a new activity or training regime.
b) When learning a new sport.
c) When needing a positive perspective on those days when it is difficult to get started exercising.
d) When facing any new situation that needs a positive perspective.

Celebration Parties

For several years, I hosted a celebration party to celebrate my successes with the people in my support network. I had these parties in August after the last triathlon of the summer. In attendance were people from all parts of my life: family, business friends, college friends and personal friends. One year, some of our college friends from Wisconsin came and saw me finish a triathlon in the rain and then came to the party. Of course, Mickey, my best friend, and Keith were there too. Most of the people knew me before I started my fitness journey so they were thrilled to celebrate my success.

Documentation

Later, I started another list of just my fitness milestones. These included events or accomplishments that were important to me, such as buying a swimming suit without a skirt or running in shorts for the first time. I documented the first time I went to the Y and swam with other people around. My fitness journey list includes many milestones and accomplishments during the first few years of my fitness journey. They are all worth celebrating.

Pins

I also celebrate my fitness accomplishments with pins.

My first pin was a suggestion from my mom. She encouraged me to celebrate completing my first race, the Rice Street Mile. This pin has a

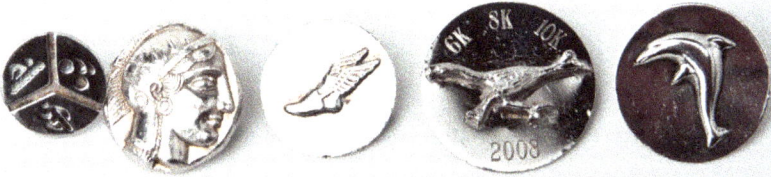

My Pins

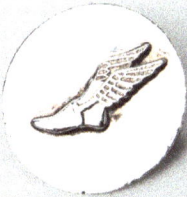

Finishing my first race: The Rice
Street Mile

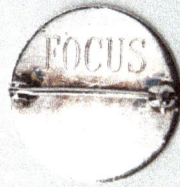

Back of the Mercury pin

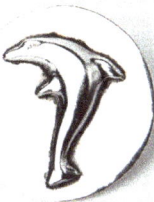

Finishing my first triathlon:
Alexandria

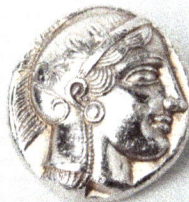

Athena Pin

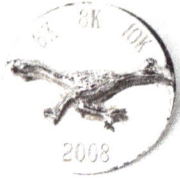

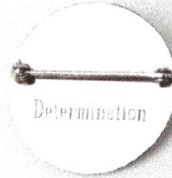

Roadrunner pin and back: Determination

running shoe with wings on the front signifying the Roman god Mercury and the word FOCUS on the back. This is because Keith taught me to focus on what I can do, not on what I can't.

My second pin has a dolphin on it to celebrate completing my first triathlon. When I was struggling to learn to swim more effectively, I tried to swim like a dolphin, which glides through the water effortlessly.

My third pin is a replica of an ancient Greek coin with an Athena on it. This is to celebrate that I lost 100 pounds. In sports events, an Athena is a woman who weighs more than 145 pounds. I will always be an Athena, but I will be a fit, healthy, balanced one.

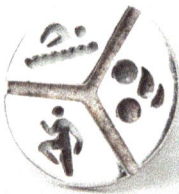

Run/Bike/Swim pin commemorating
first Olympic triathlon

The fourth pin is a roadrunner, because when I'm running, I try to run as fast as a roadrunner (Beep! Beep!). On the front it says, *6K, 8K,* and *10K 2008.* On the back it says: *Determination.* It takes a lot of determination to finish those longer distance races.

The fifth pin has the Run/Bike/Swim symbols of a triathlon. It celebrates the completion of my first Olympic Distance triathlon in August 2011.

New Bike

One early goal that I set for myself was that, when I reached my goal weight, I would get a new bike. In 2012, I decided that, although I could still lose more weight, I would treat myself to a new set of wheels.

Again, my brother-in-law Jeffrey Burton helped me pick out a new one. It is a Specialized Vita Pro—a red and white beauty! It has an aluminum frame and narrow tires, and I just love riding it. Now that I am doing more destination events, I have a bike box and take my precious bike with me. For local events, it rides in a bike rack on my husband's car. It is not a true triathlon bike with aero bars, but I have had some great rides on it.

Tattoos

This may be an off-beat way to celebrate, but why not get a tattoo? My son Ben and his wife, Sara, have had tattoos for years and periodically get more to memorialize a lost friend or a beloved grandfather. I have seen athletes at triathlons with swim-bike-run tattoos or "70.5" to signify an Ironman distance event.

With that in mind, I am considering commemorating my fitness journey with a small tattoo on my calf—a phoenix, the symbol of rebirth. This could be my way to celebrate my personal fitness journey in a different, more public way.

Display Space in Basement

Another way to celebrate my accomplishments is a display space in my basement workout area. I have a shelf for three-dimensional prizes and participation objects. I also display the box, mugs, coffee cups, plaques and plates I have received over the years.

Another type of reward is a ribbon. Sometimes you get a ribbon for crossing the finish line. Other times you get a ribbon for placing in your age group. These are proudly displayed on a rack with "Swim, Bike, Run, Play" at the top.

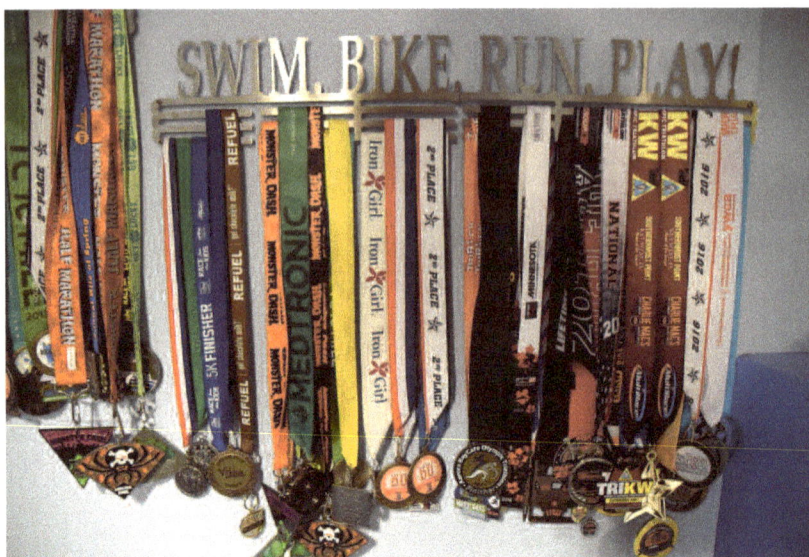

Basement Display Rack

Annual Books

Each year, I keep a scrapbook of my events. For each event, I include registration information, event emails, my racing bib, results and photographs. It is a great way to document my events and remember my firsts—whether it was my first race or first triathlon of the year, or if it led to a personal best. Many of the photos illustrating this book have come from these volumes.

When I became Fitness Person of the Year in 2013, these books were featured in the video.

Fitness Person of the Year

In 2013, I was honored by the YWCA of St. Paul as the Fitness Person of the Year. I celebrated with many members of my informal support team, including my husband, my mother, siblings, sons and many friends. I was also especially pleased that Keith and Marq Stankowski were there.

Part of that presentation was a video about how the Y was part of my fitness journey. The link is:

https://www.youtube.com/watch?v=rxTMq7QygYc.

In this video, you will see how determination, along with supportive people and groups, make a huge difference in goal achievement.

I also received a gift card which I used to buy a bike box, so I could transport my beautiful Specialized bicycle to events. Every time I use the bike box, I remember how I earned it and all of the wonderful people who have cheered me on over the years.

Summary

The important part about celebration is that I do it often. I celebrate in ways that bring me pleasure or help me to remember what is positive in my life.

In business, I have used this with my clients. One person who had a part-time business became profitable for the first time. I suggested she celebrate that, even though the dollar amount was small. Celebrating success encourages more success.

Obviously, I need to celebrate in a way that won't undermine my triumphs. I always tease Keith by telling him I am going to celebrate not eating fast food for six months with a Trademark Protected cheeseburger!

Other tangible symbols could be charms on a bracelet, trophies, a display of winning ribbons from races, and wearing your race shirt. I get ideas to inspire others, or gift ideas for family and friends who are part of the support group.

There are many ways to applaud myself. Celebrations can be public or private, something that I want to share with the world or something private, known only by me. However I celebrate my accomplishments, I celebrate them proudly.

Chapter 7

The Importance of Knowing My Body

One benefit of my fitness journey that I never anticipated is that I have learned more about my body. It started when I was learning my first stretches and strength training with Keith, when he would explain which muscles he was training and how different muscles worked together. For example, I had difficulty using my triceps muscles, and Keith tried many different exercises to find one that would allow progress without injuries.

Massage led to better understanding where I was tight and how exercise could help. I also learned how stress affected my body. For example, I carry a lot of stress in my feet. My profession of mobile accounting leads to a lot of driving, and my feet were definitely under stress. Reflexology helped, and, as I transition into retirement, driving less has helped my feet. I no longer walk barefoot on hard floors. The padded slippers I wear are much kinder to my feet.

After my surgery, my abdomen was tight, and this became a new place where I would feel stress. Again, I learned to listen to my body.

Yoga, and later Pilates, taught me balance and a new appreciation of my strong, physically fit body. I was never a yoga star, but I learned a new appreciation and knowledge of my body.

Again, the process of learning about my body is ongoing. Now, when I get a massage from a new therapist, I know what to ask for, and I know my body well enough to be able to communicate my needs. When I finish an event, I am proud of my active, physically fit body. I have learned how important it is to stretch each day to help keep my body limber as I age. As I look to the future, I take comfort in knowing that my body will help me communicate with health professionals, so I can receive the proper care.

Before I started my fitness journey my body was just there. The only time in the past I really paid attention to it was when I was pregnant. Now I am aware of my body in so many ways that it still amazes me.

Chapter 8

Planning for Travel

There are activities that bring together several lessons I have learned. The best example is planning for trips and vacations.

I had previously thought about time off and vacations as a way to take a vacation from my routine, but I have learned that, for me, it's not a healthy way to plan for success.

I have gone on many cruises in the last 12 years, and I have rarely gained more than 2–4 pounds. Most people gain as many as 10 pounds! My success has been because of two factors: perspective and planning.

My perspective is that a vacation is an opportunity to focus on fitness instead of taking a vacation from my goals and activities. If one of my barriers is lack of time, now I have as much time as I need to accomplish my goals. In the morning, instead of going to work, I can start with an aerobic activity or a strength training session.

Instead of attacking a buffet as if it is a race, I can look at it as an opportunity to try some new healthy foods that I haven't tried before or don't have readily available. This is an opportunity to eat fresh mango and pineapple and have a salad with an unusual vegetable from another part of the world. Another trick for a buffet is to eat salad and fruit first. Then I limit myself to one plate of food. At home I don't eat plate after plate of food, so why should I when I'm on vacation?

When planning for a vacation, if I have a choice of hotels, I find one that has a fitness center. I proactively check the hours and the available equipment on the hotel's website, so I can plan my activities accordingly.

Another option, if I can't choose the hotel, is to Google health clubs in the vicinity. I can often get day passes for a reasonable fee. I belong to a YWCA, and sometimes, there may be complimentary privileges available. Again, I proactively check it out ahead of time, so I can plan my workouts even while out of town.

I can also plan when attending a business conference. When I get the program booklet and plan for sessions I will be attending, I plan my workouts also. This is also a time to be flexible with my routines. Two half-hour sessions may be easier to accomplish than an hour. By being mindful and focused on what I can do, I may get more business accomplished as well.

SECTION THREE

HOW I STARTED

Day	Date	Total Minutes	Running Minutes	% Running Total	Enter Goal	Exercises	Day1	Day 2	Day 3	Percent Complete
PFS, Inc.	Weekly Running Percentage and workout compliance form 2008					WEEK 1				
Steps per minute: 180										
Weekly Goal: 180 minutes per						completed days of the week-enter 1 if completed or 0 if not				
						Date	10-Jun	11-Jun	14-Jun	
						Day of week	Tues	We	Sat	
SA				#DIV/0!		Squat	1	1	1	100.00%
SU				#DIV/0!		Chest	1	1	1	100.00%
M				#DIV/0!		Leg Extension	1	1	1	100.00%
T				#DIV/0!		Lat/Row	1	1	1	100.00%
W				#DIV/0!		Hip Flexor	1	1	1	100.00%
R				#DIV/0!		Overhead press	1	1	1	100.00%
F				#DIV/0!		Leg curl	1	1	1	100.00%
						Up Row	1	1	1	100.00%
SA				#DIV/0!		Abduction	0	0	1	33.33%
SU				#DIV/0!		Adduction	0	0	1	33.33%
M				#DIV/0!		Tricep ext.	1	0	0	33.33%
T				#DIV/0!		Calves	1	0	1	66.67%
W				#DIV/0!		Bicep Curl	1	0	1	66.67%
R				#DIV/0!		Abdominals	1	1	1	100.00%
F				#DIV/0!		Back Extension	1	0	1	66.67%
						completed days of the week-enter 1 if completed or 0 if not				
						stretches	Day1	Day 2	Day 3	Percent Complete
						Palms-up	1	1	1	100.00%
						Palms-down	1	1	1	100.00%
						Runners-floor	1	1	1	100.00%
						Outer Hip-floor	1	1	1	100.00%
						Groin-feet wide	1	1	1	100.00%
						Hip Flexor/Quad	1	1	1	100.00%
						Hamstring	1	1	1	100.00%
						Calf-facing	1	1	1	100.00%
						Tricep	1	1	1	100.00%
						Chest	1	1	1	100.00%
						Shoulder	1	1	1	100.00%
						Neck-all sides	1	1	1	100.00%

2008 chart to keep track of compliance

Chapter 9

Planning Documentation and Accountability

Planning/Diagramming/Documentation

Fail to Plan—Plan to Fail.

I learned that I needed to plan my workouts and my meals and that there are many methods to accomplish this. I prefer to use spreadsheets because I can just duplicate them each week and fill in the blanks.

At the beginning of my fitness journey, documenting my workouts was part of the compliance that Keith wanted to see. He wanted to see that I would work out the prescribed amount of time per day. It was also important for him to see my progress in learning different stretches. Here are three examples of my documentation.

From 2008: (See chart to left)

Now, diagramming my workouts is part of my weekly planning. I plan my clients, my training, my personal life and my workouts. I don't always follow the exact plan because "Life is what happens when you're making other plans," but most weeks, I do achieve my fitness goals. Keith challenges me to complete

90% of my weekly plan, so I can progress through the macrotraining cycle. Again, I use a spreadsheet that includes my heart rate during training.

Another type of documentation has been to keep records of all my events. Each year, I catalog my events chronologically in a three-ring binder, listing all events, the time it took to complete them and related mementos or photos.

I also summarize my accomplishments. As of April 2018, here are my results:

Summary to April 1, 2018:

	Percent		
	1.14%	2	1 Mile
	43.18%	76	5Ks
	0.57%	1	6K
	0.57%	1	3.9 Mile
	1.14%	2	4 mile
	3.98%	7	8K
	11.93%	21	10K
	0.57%	1	14K
	3.41%	6	10 mile
	1.14%	2	Half marathon
	0.57%	1	Indoor triathlon
	17.61%	31	Sprint triathlons
	1.14%	2	Long sprint triathlons
	2.84%	5	Olympic distance triathlons
	3.98%	7	Duathlons
	2.27%	4	Bike only (2 duathlons, 2 triathlons)
	3.98%	7	DNF- Did not Finish
Total:	100.00%	176	
	21.59%	38	All triathlons

Formal Fitness Testing

For several years, once a month, Keith documented certain exercises so I could see my progress. These included pushups, a sit-and-reach test, an aerobic step test and several others. Later, after Keith expanded my testing, he added in many more flexibility and motor firing tests. This also helped him to design strength training regimens that would properly meet my needs.

Here is an example of Keith's fitness testing for me: (See diagram on next page.)

Documentation

Documentation of diet is important, and I explained the importance of documenting my food when I was describing my nutrition journey in Chapter 1.

Another type of documentation is a Periodization, which is also described in Chapter 1. I explained that Keith had me working on fixed periodization schedules and on variable schedules. Here are examples of the intelligent documentation he trained me to use: (Chart on page 83.)

Keith also taught me to use documentation for better stress management. Here is an example of the documentation I used to monitor and manage stress. We detailed specific factors to clarify the effects of individual stress contributors.

Stress Monitoring Document

Documentation has been an essential part of my success. I found that it can be used for celebration—I achieved my goals and now I can get that new workout outfit I have been eyeing. It has also been helpful when I'm not meeting my benchmarks and has motivated me to get help from my formal and informal support teams. When I take time to review my documentation, I can see how far I've come. It's uplifting and encouraging—something we all need.

Name	test	Comp	test	Comp	test	Comp		MHR	207	RHR	
								Age			
Date:				0				Est. MHR	207		
Height (inches)								HRR	207		
RHR				0				LHHR	HHRR	MHHR	
Weight (lbs.)				0				93.15	165.6	129.375	
BC%				0		Goal:					
Fat lbs.				0		Goal:					
W/H ratio				0		Goal:					
Post step HR				0		Goal:					
Push-ups				0		Goal:					
Sit-ups				0		Goal:					
sit/reach				0		Goal:					
r-shoulder				0		Goal:					
l-shoulder				0		Goal:					
BMI							0	0	0		
Date:	LEFT	RIGHT	GOAL	S = SHORT							
Leg Length											
ASIS											
Ilium Rocking											
Hams			90								
Piriformis											
Adductors											
Trapezius											
Levator Scapulae											
CCP: S = SHORT B = FASCIAL BIAS	LEFT	RIGHT									
Lumbo-Sacral (L-S)											
Thoraco-Lumbar (T-L)											
Cervico-Thoracic (C-T)											
Atlanto-Occipital (A-O)											
PRONE:	LEFT	RIGHT	GOAL								
PSOAS-Prone			8								
Rectus Femoris-Prone			8								
IF jt. capsule-Prone			4								
FIRING ORDER	LEFT	RIGHT	GOAL								
Hamstrings			1								
Gluteus Maximus			2								
Contralateral Erectors			3								
Ipsilateral Erectors			4								
SIDELYING	LEFT	RIGHT	GOAL								
Gluteus Medius			1								
TFL			2								
Quadratus Lumborum			3								
SHOULDER & NECK: STANDING	LEFT	RIGHT	GOAL								
shoulder abduction-frontal plane			180								
horizontal external rotation-humerus			180								
Neck rotation-wall			90								
axial rotation-wall			90								
standing hip flexion-wall			90								
side bend-wall			60								

Triathlon Training Plan for a 13 week cycle-Spreadsheet calculations
Training plan for Olympic Triathlon
Projected year hours to train   400

Four week cycle	1	2	3	4	5	6	7
Training Stage	Base	Base	Intensity	Intensity	Peak	Peak	Race
Week numbers	1 thru 4	5 thru 8	9 thru 12	13 thru 13	17 thru 20	21 thru 22	23 thru 26
Actual dates							
% of yearly hours	8%	8%	8%	2%	0%	0%	0%
Hours/cycle	32	32	32	8	0	0	0

Week number	1	2	3	4	5	6	7	8	9	10	11	12	13	14	15	16	17	18	19	20	21	22	23	24	25
Periodization	25%	25%	25%	25%	25%	25%	25%	25%	25%	25%	25%	25%	100%	0%	0%	0%	0%	0%	0%	0%	0%	0%	0%	0%	0%
Hours/week	8.0	8.0	8.0	8.0	8.0	8.0	8.0	8.0	8.0	8.0	8.0	8.0	8.0	0.0	0.0	0.0	0.0	0.0	0.0	0.0	0.0	0.0	0.0	0.0	0.0

Below: Total minutes per week of each SERIOUS component

	1	2	3	4	5	6	7	8	9	10	11	12	13	14	15	16	17	18	19	20	21	22	23	24	25
Speed - Wkly Tot	0	0	0	0	0	0	0	0	24	24	24	24	24	0	0	0	0	0	0	0	0	0	0	0	0
Swim	0	0	0	0	0	0	0	0	0	0	0	0	0	0	0	0	0	0	0	0	0	0	0	0	0
Bike	0	0	0	0	0	0	0	0	12	12	12	12	12	0	0	0	0	0	0	0	0	0	0	0	0
Run	0	0	0	0	0	0	0	0	12	12	12	12	12	0	0	0	0	0	0	0	0	0	0	0	0
Endurance	72	72	72	72	72	72	72	72	72	72	72	72	72	0	0	0	0	0	0	0	0	0	0	0	0
Swim	14	14	14	14	14	14	14	14	14	14	14	14	14	0	0	0	0	0	0	0	0	0	0	0	0
Bike	36	36	36	36	36	36	36	36	36	36	36	36	36	0	0	0	0	0	0	0	0	0	0	0	0
Run	22	22	22	22	22	22	22	22	22	22	22	22	22	0	0	0	0	0	0	0	0	0	0	0	0
Race/Pace	0	0	0	0	0	0	0	0	24	24	24	24	48	0	0	0	0	0	0	0	0	0	0	0	0
Swim	0	0	0	0	0	0	0	0	5	5	5	5	10	0	0	0	0	0	0	0	0	0	0	0	0
Bike	0	0	0	0	0	0	0	0	12	12	12	12	24	0	0	0	0	0	0	0	0	0	0	0	0
Run	0	0	0	0	0	0	0	0	7	7	7	7	14	0	0	0	0	0	0	0	0	0	0	0	0
Intervals	48	48	48	48	96	96	96	96	96	96	96	96	48	0	0	0	0	0	0	0	0	0	0	0	0
Swim	17	17	17	17	34	34	34	34	34	34	34	34	17	0	0	0	0	0	0	0	0	0	0	0	0
Bike	17	17	17	17	34	34	34	34	34	34	34	34	17	0	0	0	0	0	0	0	0	0	0	0	0
Run	14	14	14	14	29	29	29	29	29	29	29	29	14	0	0	0	0	0	0	0	0	0	0	0	0
Overdistance	264	264	264	264	264	264	264	264	216	216	216	216	240	0	0	0	0	0	0	0	0	0	0	0	0
Swim	53	53	53	53	53	53	53	53	43	43	43	43	48	0	0	0	0	0	0	0	0	0	0	0	0
Bike	132	132	132	132	132	132	132	132	108	108	108	108	120	0	0	0	0	0	0	0	0	0	0	0	0
Run	79	79	79	79	79	79	79	79	65	65	65	65	72	0	0	0	0	0	0	0	0	0	0	0	0
Up/Vertical	0	0	0	0	0	0	0	0	0	0	0	0	0	0	0	0	0	0	0	0	0	0	0	0	0
Swim	0	0	0	0	0	0	0	0	0	0	0	0	0	0	0	0	0	0	0	0	0	0	0	0	0
Bike	0	0	0	0	0	0	0	0	0	0	0	0	0	0	0	0	0	0	0	0	0	0	0	0	0
Run	0	0	0	0	0	0	0	0	0	0	0	0	0	0	0	0	0	0	0	0	0	0	0	0	0
Strength	96	96	96	96	48	48	48	48	48	48	48	48	48	0	0	0	0	0	0	0	0	0	0	0	0

Fixed Periodization Schedule

Triathlon Training Plan for a 12.5 week cycle-Spreadsheet calculations
Training plan for Olympic Triathlon
Projected year hours to train   450

Four week cycle	1	2	3	4	5	6	7
Training Stage	Base	Base	Intensity	Intensity	Peak	Peak	Race
Week numbers	1 thru 4	5 thru 8	9 thru 12	14 thru 16	17 thru 20	21 thru 24	25 thru 26
Actual dates							
% of yearly hours	0%	0%	0%	6%	8%	8%	3%
Hours/cycle	0	0	0	27	36	36	13

Week number	1	2	3	4	5	6	7	8	9	10	11	12	13	14	15	16	17	18	19	20	21	22	23	24	25	26
Periodization	23%	27%	31%	19%	23%	27%	31%	19%	23%	26%	29%	22%	0%	26%	29%	22%	23%	26%	29%	22%	23%	26%	29%	22%	70%	30%
Hours/week	0.0	0.0	0.0	0.0	0.0	0.0	0.0	0.0	0.0	0.0	0.0	0.0	0.0	7.0	7.8	5.9	8.3	9.4	10.4	7.9	8.3	9.4	10.4	7.9	9.1	3.9

Below: Total minutes per week of each SERIOUS component

	1	2	3	4	5	6	7	8	9	10	11	12	13	14	15	16	17	18	19	20	21	22	23	24	25	26
Speed - Wkly Tot	0	0	0	0	0	0	0	0	0	0	0	0	0	21	23	18	25	28	31	24	25	28	31	24	27	12
Swim	0	0	0	0	0	0	0	0	0	0	0	0	0	0	0	0	0	0	0	0	0	0	0	0	0	0
Bike	0	0	0	0	0	0	0	0	0	0	0	0	0	11	12	9	12	14	16	12	12	14	16	12	14	6
Run	0	0	0	0	0	0	0	0	0	0	0	0	0	11	12	9	12	14	16	12	12	14	16	12	14	6
Endurance	0	0	0	0	0	0	0	0	0	0	0	0	0	63	70	53	75	84	94	71	50	56	63	48	55	23
Swim	0	0	0	0	0	0	0	0	0	0	0	0	0	13	14	11	15	17	19	14	10	11	13	10	11	5
Bike	0	0	0	0	0	0	0	0	0	0	0	0	0	32	36	27	37	42	47	36	25	28	31	24	27	12
Run	0	0	0	0	0	0	0	0	0	0	0	0	0	19	21	16	22	25	28	21	15	17	19	14	16	7
Race/Pace	0	0	0	0	0	0	0	0	0	0	0	0	0	42	47	36	50	56	63	48	75	84	94	71	82	35
Swim	0	0	0	0	0	0	0	0	0	0	0	0	0	8	9	7	10	11	13	10	15	17	19	14	16	7
Bike	0	0	0	0	0	0	0	0	0	0	0	0	0	21	23	18	25	28	31	24	37	42	47	36	41	18
Run	0	0	0	0	0	0	0	0	0	0	0	0	0	13	14	11	15	17	19	14	22	25	28	21	25	11
Intervals	0	0	0	0	0	0	0	0	0	0	0	0	0	42	47	36	50	56	63	48	50	56	63	48	55	23
Swim	0	0	0	0	0	0	0	0	0	0	0	0	0	15	16	12	17	20	22	17	17	20	22	17	19	8
Bike	0	0	0	0	0	0	0	0	0	0	0	0	0	15	16	12	17	20	22	17	17	20	22	17	19	8
Run	0	0	0	0	0	0	0	0	0	0	0	0	0	13	14	11	15	17	19	14	15	17	19	14	16	7
Overdistance	0	0	0	0	0	0	0	0	0	0	0	0	0	211	235	178	248	281	313	238	248	281	313	238	273	117
Swim	0	0	0	0	0	0	0	0	0	0	0	0	0	42	47	36	50	56	63	48	50	56	63	48	55	23
Bike	0	0	0	0	0	0	0	0	0	0	0	0	0	105	117	89	124	140	157	119	124	140	157	119	137	59
Run	0	0	0	0	0	0	0	0	0	0	0	0	0	63	70	53	75	84	94	71	75	84	94	71	82	35
Up/Vertical	0	0	0	0	0	0	0	0	0	0	0	0	0	0	0	0	0	0	0	0	0	0	0	0	0	0
Swim	0	0	0	0	0	0	0	0	0	0	0	0	0	0	0	0	0	0	0	0	0	0	0	0	0	0
Bike	0	0	0	0	0	0	0	0	0	0	0	0	0	0	0	0	0	0	0	0	0	0	0	0	0	0
Run	0	0	0	0	0	0	0	0	0	0	0	0	0	0	0	0	0	0	0	0	0	0	0	0	0	0
Strength	0	0	0	0	0	0	0	0	0	0	0	0	0	42	47	36	50	56	63	48	50	56	63	48	55	23

Variable Periodization Schedule

Date of Consultation	22-Jun	27-Jun	4-Jul	11-Jul		
Factor						
1 Job	(3.0)	(3.0)	(2.0)	(2.0)		
2 Driving		(2.0)	1.0	(1.0)		
3	(1.0)	0.5	1.0	0.0		
4	0.5	0.5	0.0	0.0		
	(0.5)					
5 Person of Interest	(0.5)		0.5	1.0		
	(1.0)	(1.5)	(1.0)	(1.0)		
6	(2.0)	(1.5)	(2.0)	(2.0)		
7 Nutrition	1.0	0.5	1.0	1.0		
8	0.5	0.0				
9 Fitness Training	1.0	2.0	2.0	2.5		
10 Volunteering		(1.0)	1.0	1.0		
Total	(5.0)	(5.5)	1.5	(0.5)		

Stress Monitoring Document

Chapter 10

Barriers and How I Overcome Them

One of the reasons I wrote this book was because many friends and acquaintances said, "You are such an inspiration, but I could never do what you did." The truth is that everyone has the ability to make changes in their life, but it takes work and determination. In this next section are some of those, "But I never could because…" comments and my replies, using the lessons I have learned.

1. I don't have the time.
When I started, Keith had me do three minutes of aerobics a day. I don't know anyone who doesn't have three minutes. His only expectation was that each week I would add a minute per day for that new week. Then, when I reached 30 minutes a day, I could have a day off.

The point is that through diagramming and planning, I can find time to exercise. See Chapter 9.

2. I can't afford a trainer.
I cannot afford not to use one. I found a professional with the right training and experience to help me with my journey. I cannot tell you how much

having the right trainer has saved me in other costs such as medications, insurance premiums, doctor visits and unnecessary pain. I can only express how much joy and ambition I now have every day.

Ask for a gift certificate for your birthday or for a holiday present.

I see having my trainer as an investment in my health. A healthier me will need fewer medications and doctor visits. By taking good care of myself, I will also be in better shape physically and mentally to take good care of the important people in my life.

3. I don't like to work out at a gym, or I am embarrassed at how I look when working out.

I have never needed to join a gym. I worked out of my home or at my trainer's studio. I have never needed expensive equipment. My first set of equipment was resistance bands that cost less than $10 each. I later added a trampoline that cost about $40. I bought used equipment at second-hand stores and garage sales. A gym or health club membership is not required for excellent health and fitness.

Here is a picture of two of our grandchildren on the elliptical in our basement room that is used for both working out and as a play space for our four grandchildren.

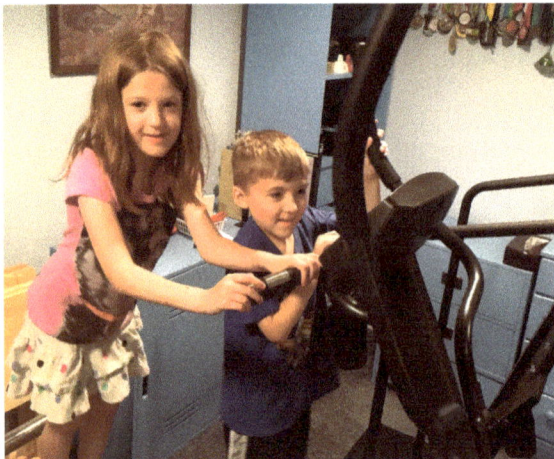

Macy and Emmett on my elliptical machine

Here are pictures of me using equipment in my basement workout area. The mirrors on the wall help with my routines by reminding me of proper stance and posture while working out.

My exercise room is my happy place!

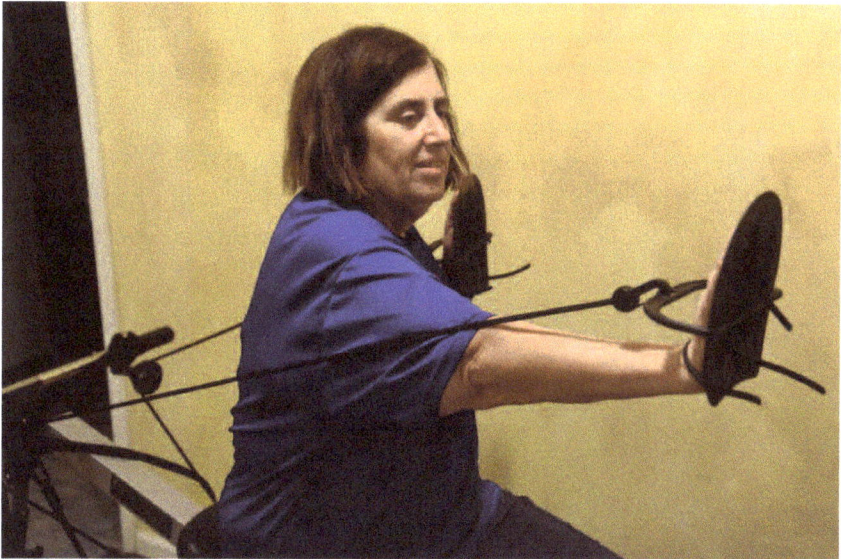

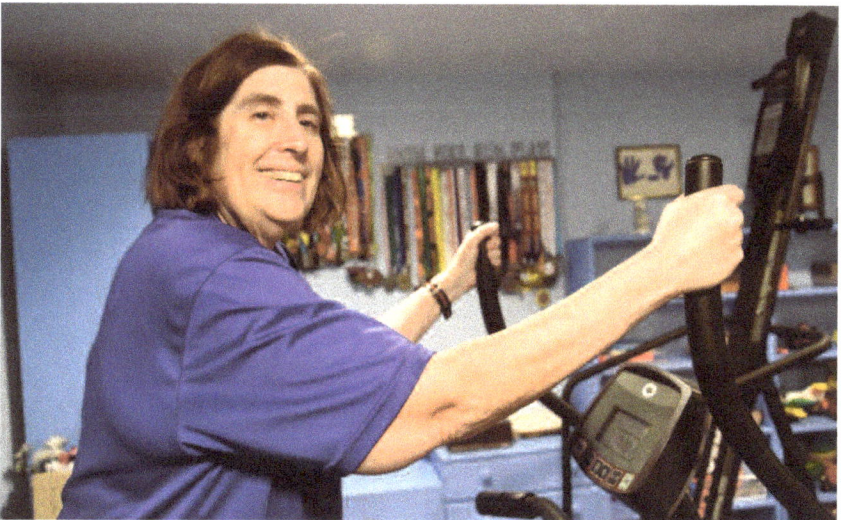

Chapter 11

My Continuing Journey

Any life journey is going to have ups and downs, waxing and waning. I understand that if I stick to my core plan, the bumps in the road will not be detours but learning experiences.

Friends have asked me how I got started. It all began with setting goals as I explained in Chapter 4, then documentation as in Chapter 9, and accountability. I have found that working with a professional on accountability has led to the greatest success.

This book ends at the beginning of 2018, but my journey has not ended. I am still working with my trainer, Keith Gosline; and since he has moved to the Dominican Republic, we now train together every six or eight weeks. We continue our weekly accountability sessions and, when we meet in person, he reviews my progress and sets new goals and regimens.

A longer-term goal is to complete a triathlon with one of my grandchildren. Since Macy is ten, Emmett seven, Evelyn four and Asher one at the time of this writing, it won't be happening soon, but won't it be great!

Another of my goals is to be the oldest person to complete a triathlon. In Minnesota, I am one of the older women still completing triathlons. Since Bob Powers is 92, this is definitely a long-term goal!

But my journey is not just about events. I want to be active and healthy and live a splendid life. I also want you, my readers, to feel empowered to begin your own fitness journeys. Let me know if this book has helped you to find inspiration and motivation within yourself. It can be done!

There are no quick fixes! How did I change from the woman who was seriously obese and out of shape to an athlete who exercises purposefully, competes in multiple events each year and has a healthy relationship with food? It did not happen overnight. I did not move from a sedentary lifestyle to that of a healthy athlete in 60 days. It took time, determination and support. The quick version of my journey so far is this:

In January of 2006, I was an overweight, middle-aged, sedentary accountant. My life coach, Jeanne Heald, suggested I work with a personal trainer, so I met with Keith Gosline of Personal Fitness Systems in St. Paul on January 23rd and started working out on January 30th.

That decision has transformed me. First, I have become fit. I started with three minutes of aerobics a day and now do 50+ minutes, five days a week. With a focused exercise regimen and healthy eating habits, I have gone from 346 to about 180 pounds. I trained with Keith and participated in over 176 different events, in a variety of locations. I am now an athlete.

I have been transformed in three ways:
1. I have new confidence that I can accomplish my goals. If I can go from sedentary to fit, what else can I accomplish?
2. I now get as much pleasure from physical accomplishments as I had gotten in the past from academic degrees or from successes with my accounting clients.
3. I have experienced a marvelous change in attitude. I now focus on what I can do, not on what I cannot.

I wish the same results, and even better, for you!

How do you start? Set a goal that is measurable, achievable and flexible. Have fun! Become the active, happy, fit person that you were meant to be.

What is most important?

- **Have a plan.**
- **Keep a positive attitude** as there will be missteps, lack of progress, and even DNFs. But when you look back, you will realize that you have accomplished more than you ever thought possible.
- **Document.** This will help you recognize your progress and have information with which to make changes.
- **Celebrate** your accomplishments, your perseverance and your successes.

Remember this is a journey for the rest of your life!

Lindsay B. Nauen
St. Paul, Minnesota
Spring 2018

Acknowledgments

To Members of My Formal and Informal Support Teams

Formal Support Team—Fitness Journey

Jeanne Heald, life coach, who recommended that I get a trainer.

Dr. John Beecher, my personal physician, who gave me the medical okay to start training.

Ann Short, my massage therapist, who weekly keeps me ready for my workouts and events.

Dr. William Katsiyiannis, my cardiologist, who monitors by PVCs so I can train at high intensity.

Dr. Emily Fields, my psychologist, who has helped me understand I have the power and ability to change myself, and not other people.

And of course—Keith Gosline, my trainer, who started this journey with me and has supported me throughout.

Formal Support Team—Fitness Journey Book

Gloria Russell, my editor, who always believed in me.

Sue Stein, my book designer, for her creative ideas and design.

Sun Lund and David Grupa, my photographers, who have created visuals to enhance this book.

Keith Gosline, trainer and friend, whose helpful comments and commentary have enhanced this book.

Informal Support Team

Marq Stankowski—As the first member of my informal support team, he taught me balance and has grown from mentor to dear friend.

Richard—My husband of 43 years has been an enthusiastic supporter of my fitness journey. He even started a journey of his own and has become great at half marathons.

Our family—Our sons, Noah and Ben, their wives, Brianna and Sara, and our grandchildren, Macy, Emmett, Evelyn and Asher, are all part of my support team. One of my goals is to participate in a triathlon with a grandchild!

My family—My mother Joyce, brother Charlie, sisters Varda and Elinor, have all supported me. They have been at some events and we have done others together. My brothers-in-law, Johnny and Jeffrey, and my nieces and nephew, Rachel, Hannah, Zoe and Henry, have also encouraged and supported me. Also, to my one and only sister-in-law P.J. Pofahl, I appreciate your support.

Extended family—I have a super group of what we call FC. These include first cousins, their spouses, children and grandchildren. Also included are an aunt and various other cousin relationships.

Best friend—Mickey Levinger is that best friend every woman needs. We started our friendship as mothers of sons, and she has supported me loyally throughout my journey.

Friends—My friends have been so supportive and interested in my journey. I know I have years more to enjoy these relationships I have chosen.

Gary Westlund—Founder and President at Charities Challenge, also an ACSM coach, has been a long-time encourager.

Sean Truman & Jerry McNeil—Friends who have encouraged me on my journey since the beginning.

My indoor cycling instructors at the YWCA of St. Paul, who helped me enjoy group exercises and have always been interested in and supportive of my journey.

Of special note are our Madison friends, Dennis, Matt and Jane. They have traveled to see me participate in events and attended the celebration when I was named Fitness Person of the Year.

To all of you: thank you for your love and support!

ABOUT THE TRAINER

Keith Gosline, ACSM EP-C, CKTP, CMAT

Keith Gosline is a well-rounded, health-conscious movement and fitness expert. Keith provides what he terms a "continuum of care" of functional, palpatory and visual testing, myoskeletal align-ment therapy (MAT), kinesio taping, and a progressive and customized exercise training plan to get each person from "pain to play."

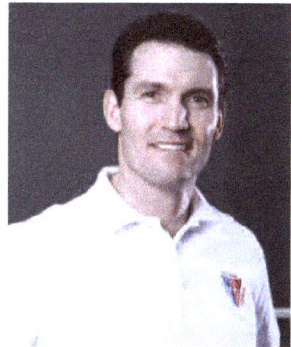

Keith's mission is family fitness. He teaches his clients how family members can support one another with the same knowledge and same system of progressive training instruction as each person travels through their fitness and wellness journey.

"Just because we can, does not mean we should" is a quote Keith likes to use with his clients to start the process of change in their daily lives. Keith demonstrates how and why our daily dysfunctional motor patterns and habits of improper sitting, standing, sleeping, walking, exercising and running can promote pain, inflammation, joint degradation, poor work and training performance, and poor health. Conversely, he teaches how and why we are designed to move through his continuum of care.

Keith is the Founder and Owner of Gosline-MAPP, SRL in Santo Domingo, Dominican Republic. MAPP signifies Myoskeletal Alignment for Pain and Performance. He started his fitness business in Fargo, North Dakota in 1992, incorporated in 1997, and moved the corporation to Minnesota in 2003. In December of 2014, Keith moved to the Dominican Republic.

Keith has a Bachelor of Applied Science degree in Exercise, Fitness, and Sports Science from the Minnesota State University Moorhead. He is a certified advanced myoskeletal alignment practitioner (CMAT), certified kinesio taping practitioner (CKTP), and American College of Sports Medicine-certified exercise physiologist (ACSM EP-C). He has also been trained and certified in reflexology and massage therapy.

As a bilingual fitness and manual therapy practitioner, Keith has made a career of providing professional guidance based on an integration of disciplines in physical sciences (human biomechanics, anatomy, physiology, etc.) combined with large doses of compassion and encouragement.

You can connect with Keith Gosline at Gosline-MAPP, Calle Paseo de los Locutores # 58, Esq. Padre Emiliano Tardif. Tercer Piso, Suite 310-B, Evaristo Morales, Santo Domingo, D.N. (Frente a la Casa de la Anunciación, en el Edificio donde está el Golds Gym), also by WhatsApp or phone 829-424-8014, or by connecting on LinkedIn at:

https://www.linkedin.com/in/keith-gosline-mapp/

ABOUT THE AUTHOR

Lindsay B. Nauen, MBA

Lindsay B. Nauen was born in Sioux Falls, South Dakota where she attended Washington High School and developed her love for education and continual learning.

In 1972, she earned her B.A. degree in psychology and, in 1974, earned an MLS degree, both from the University of Wisconsin–Madison. Her graduate work in history was at Temple University in Philadelphia, and, in 1988, she received an MBA with an accounting concentration from the University of Minnesota, Carlson School of Management.

Lindsay's first professional career was as an archivist and included positions in Madison, WI, Mt. Vernon, NY, Philadelphia, PA and Pierre, SD. She also worked as a librarian for Minnehaha County, SD.

In 1988, after receiving her MBA, she started her second career, in accounting, which included responsibilities as the Business Administrator of a private school before starting her own business, Nauen Mobile Accounting, in 1993. After a successful, two-decade career at Nauen Mobile Accounting assisting business owners with personalized accounting services, she sold the business to Pinkham Tax and Accounting in 2014. Lindsay continues to work part-time with the new owner, Nate Pinkham.

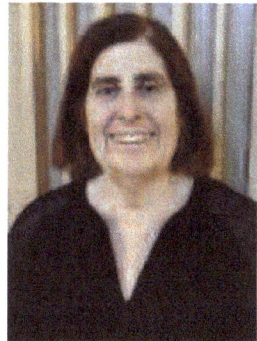

Lindsay has been married to Richard Weil since 1975. They have two sons: Noah, born in 1980, and Ben, born in 1982. Their family expanded with Ben's marriage to Sara Stadke in 2006 and Noah's marriage to Brianna Blaser in 2010. Noah and Brianna have two children: Evelyn (2014) and Asher (2017). Ben and Sara also have two children: Macy (2007) and Emmett (2010). It's a joyful occasion when they can all be together.

Acknowledging the fact that she was severely overweight and had limited physical capabilities, Lindsay began her fitness journey in 2006 which transformed her in so many delightful, healthful and unexpected ways. She is now an athlete participating in a variety of events each year and often travels with her husband, Richard, or other family members, for fun fitness destination events. Lindsay also enjoys reading, bridge and playing games. She lives in St. Paul, Minnesota and appreciates the beauty of its seasonal changes.

You can connect with Lindsay on LinkedIn at: *https://www.linkedin.com/in/lindsaynauen/*